P9-CFI-111

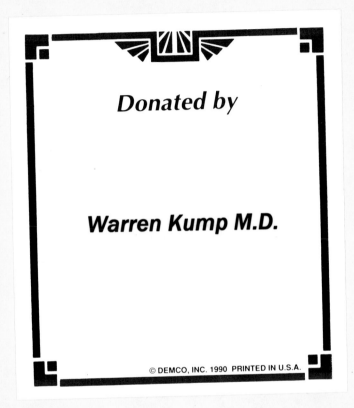

Donated by

Warren Kump M.D.

© DEMCO, INC. 1990 PRINTED IN U.S.A.

THE TEACHING HOSPITAL

Evolution and Contemporary Issues

MEDICAL LIBRARY
NORTH MEMORIAL HEALTH CARE
3800 OAKDALE AVENUE NORTH
ROBBINSDALE, MN 55422-2900

THE TEACHING HOSPITAL

EVOLUTION AND
CONTEMPORARY ISSUES

MEDICAL LIBRARY
NORTH MEMORIAL HEALTH CARE
3300 OAKDALE AVENUE NORTH
ROBBINSDALE, MN 55422-2900

Edited by John H. Knowles, M.D.

HARVARD UNIVERSITY PRESS

CAMBRIDGE, MASSACHUSETTS

1966

WZ80
K73t

© Copyright 1966
by the President and Fellows of Harvard College
All rights reserved
Distributed in Great Britain by Oxford University Press, London
Library of Congress Catalog Card Number 66-21338
Printed in the United States of America

16422

CONTENTS

FIGURES

TABLES

INTRODUCTION

John H. Knowles, M.D.

THE FIRST half of the twentieth century has witnessed rapid change in all aspects of our lives — economic, social, technological, medical, political, and so on. The inexorable advance of expanding science and technology has created a highly specialized and increasingly complex society which has made many of us strangers to the rapidly turning wheels of progress or change. The development of a *social* science and technology with which to obtain effective answers to an increasing number of social and economic problems has lagged behind. Bertrand Russell has said, "One of the troubles of our age is that habits of thought cannot change as quickly as techniques, with the result that as skill increases, wisdom fades." [1] Although Lord Russell's view is somewhat pessimistic, one could argue that the present nuclear arms race supports his contention.

I prefer Jerome Bruner's statement: "With technological advance, more things are possible, but social and technical organization is increasingly necessary to bring them off. In effect then, the sense of potency — the idea of the possible — increases in scope, but the artificer of the possible is now society rather than the individual." [2]

In the case of medicine, the American hospital has evolved from the quarantine hut of the eighteenth century

1

through the passive receptacle for the sick poor of the nineteenth century; to the present positive "health center" for all social and economic classes. Since the turn of this century, there have been remarkable changes in medical science (X-ray, blood typing, insulin, antibiotics, open heart surgery, and organ transplantation), social welfare (Social Security Act of 1935), and the financing of health services (Blue Cross; Kerr-Mills Amendment of 1960; P.L. 89–97 — Social Security Amendments of 1965, that is "Medicare"). Unfortunately, these remarkable developments have been matched by an equally remarkable lack of change in medical education and the medical profession. The hospital as health center now provides one of the best social and technical instruments available to the profession and to the community for the solution of the medical care problems of somatic, psychic, and social dis-ease, as well as the companion problems of rising costs and expectations. Unfortunately, the doctor still views the hospital as *his* host, and the public views it through the glasses of misinformation (or lack of information), fear, and financial hardship.

The hospital provides the platform where the profession meets the public. The "public" includes patients, expanding state and federal medical care plans (Hill-Burton; "Medicare"; Heart Disease, Cancer and Stroke Law), Blue Cross and commercial insurance companies, organized consumer unions, organized medicine in the form of state and national medical societies (the American Medical Association, American College of Radiology), political representatives, and so on. The hospital finds itself occupying the central position amidst these forces, some fighting for short-term selfish interest, but all looking with rising hopes and expectations to the institution. Better understanding of the hospital, its historical evolution, its present problems, and its obligatory role as a social instrument is necessary if the medical profession and the local community wish to keep the use of this instrument in their own hands. Change in all these forces which influence and shape the medical world demands that the medical curriculum change and that the profession change with it.

Dr. William H. Stewart, newly appointed Surgeon General of the United States Public Health Service, presented a major address to the participants in the White House Conference on Health, November 3, 1965. It was an eloquent and thoughtful talk, delivered with passion and of such moment and relevance to some of the issues discussed in this book that it bears repeating here in part. Dr. Stewart said:

The health services industry employed about one million people in 1940. Today its ranks are approaching three million. One out of every 25 gainfully employed persons in the United States today serves the cause of health.

How shall these forces be marshalled toward the accomplishment of our objective — the best health service, universally accessible?

To approach an answer to this enormous question, we must first look with unclouded vision at how these forces are being used today. And immediately we find that relatively little is known about what today's health workers actually do, how they spend their time, to what extent they make full use of the training they receive. Such data are urgently needed.

We must look objectively at the summit of the pyramid — the medical profession itself. What meaningful response can we devise — in terms of meeting human needs — to the challenge of specialization? Does the answer lie in further refinement of the principles of group practice? Does it lie in the conscious development of a new kind of family physician? Can we train a generalist who, like most generals, is at the top rather than the bottom of the totem pole, calling on specialists to assist him as the patient's condition demands? What

JOHN H. KNOWLES, M.D.

combination will maximize scientific benefit and minimize the loss of the human touch on which medicine is built?

We need to examine critically our current patterns of distribution of health manpower — both broadly, in terms of regions, and narrowly, in terms of urban neighborhoods and suburban complexes. Will today's trends simplify or complicate tomorrow's task of meeting health needs? If the distribution trends appear undesirable, how can we influence them?

The developments of the recent past have produced a medical culture which has been characterized as "islands of excellence in a sea of mediocrity." Is this a fair description? Are we, in our professional schools, so preoccupied with the purity of clinical excellence — as exemplified in our superequipped and superstaffed teaching hospitals — that there is nothing left over for raising the base of medical care in the broader community? Do we have educational programs that will prepare people to meet the needs of Appalachia, of Harlem, or even of Westchester County, New York?

Moreover, our influence and our clientele are world-wide. What do our schools offer for meeting the health needs of Southeast Asia? How long can the United States continue to support a position as an importer of physicians, an importer of nurses?

Year by year, our top professional personnel are being trained to perform still more complex tasks. How long can each profession afford to hang on to its simpler functions — the routine filling of a tooth, for example, or the several easily automated steps in a medical examination? How can we train the physician or dentist to make full use of the skills available in other people, freeing himself to perform only those duties for which he is uniquely qualified?

Moreover, artificial barriers separate one stratum of the health manpower pyramid from another, buttressed by such considerations as academic credits. Can we devise career ladders to permit the highly capable practical nurse to move into professional nursing, the professional nurse into medicine, the hygienst into dentistry? Wouldn't all the disciplines ultimately gain from such vertical mobility?

These questions, and many more. Questions in search of not

4

one but many answers, which will give shape and substance
to the education of health manpower.

Most important of all, these answers must come from many
sources. The great strength of our American system of health
service lies in its diversity. No single element — neither private
medicine nor academic medicine nor government — can write
the prescription and impose it on the rest of the partnership.
Nor can all the elements of the health partnership, acting
collectively, impose our answers upon the whole of society.
For health is so interwoven into the fabric of the American
culture that its ultimate design can only be determined by the
people themselves. [3]

To my mind, the Surgeon General has set the theme
for the coming years in medicine — the rational utilization
of medical manpower, the extension of the hospitals' interest to the community, and the joint effort of public and
private resources — in short, more energy devoted to the
utilization of knowledge as well as its acquisition so that
high quality medical care and prevention of disease will be
available to all Americans. This is a clear mandate for the
teaching hospital, which represents the interface where
knowledge is both acquired *and* utilized.

The primary function of the hospital, regardless of the
adjective used to designate its character, is the care of the
sick and injured of the community. An additional responsibility of the teaching hospital is the conservation and
expansion of knowledge through educational endeavor and
scientific research. In addition, prevention of disease and
active public health measures must become a central
effort.

In recent times, the cost-conscious public has challenged
the higher costs of teaching hospitals without recognizing
that the quality of patient care can be enhanced considerably in an environment of teaching. Moral and financial

5

support of these interdependent functions of care and teaching will be made available by the "public" if it understands the inseparable nature of them, and the fact that both the public's short-term and long-range interests are being served by the teaching function.

The issues of teaching, quality of patient care, and the organization and financing of such costly functions in the university-affiliated, teaching hospital were examined in a series of four lectures given at the Massachusetts General Hospital during February 1965 and sponsored jointly by the Lowell Institute. Subsequently two of the Lowell Lecturers assumed new posts. Dr. Robert J. Glaser became Vice President for Medical Affairs and Dean of the School of Medicine at Stanford University. Dr. Robert H. Ebert became Dean of the Faculty at Harvard Medical School on July 1, 1965.

It is our hope that the collection of these Lowell Lectures will lead to better understanding of the institution's problems and that enlightened interest will be reflected in wiser, more long-range decisions by the public as represented by our patients, elected political officials, representatives of third-party paying agencies and voluntary philanthropies, government agencies, and union officials, to say nothing of the medical school and university faculty, and the clinical staff of the hospital itself.

THE TEACHING HOSPITAL
AND THE MEDICAL SCHOOL

Robert J. Glaser, M.D.

THERE ARE in the United States today, according to the American Hospital Association, some 7138 hospitals. Among this large number of "registered hospitals" there is much diversity. In passing, one cannot escape the fact that all hospitals, irrespective of size and program, face serious problems of a common nature, originating to a large extent in the explosion of biomedical knowledge and the resultant ever-increasing complexity of modern medicine. Nonetheless, the contemporary issues referred to in the title of the current Lowell Lectures have to do with a very particular kind of hospital — the teaching hospital, and in directing our attention to this group of institutions, we limit ourselves to a very much smaller number.

Thus, of the 7138 hospitals listed as registered in 1964, 5684 are included in the category of short-term general hospitals. In terms of size, it can readily be seen in the list on the page following that there is a wide range represented. The data in the list indicate that 60 percent of the short-term general hospitals presently operating have 100 beds or less. Conversely, only 9 percent have more than 300 beds, and only slightly over 2 percent have 500 beds or more.

Without discussing the point in detail, one can say that the programs of the short-term general hospitals, as distinct from chronic disease institutions, vary considerably, in some measure depending on their size, but to a greater extent depending on whether or not they are involved in teaching. In general, teaching hospitals are among the larger rather than the smaller hospitals, usually having 300 beds or more.

Bed Capacities of the Short-Term General Hospitals
in the United States, 1964

Number of beds	Number of hospitals
Less than 25	627
25 – 49	1464
50 – 99	1466
100 – 199	1058
200 – 299	540
300 – 399	262
400 – 499	124
500 or over	143

Within the over-all classification of "teaching hospitals," there are various subdivisions. Thus, the Council on Medical Education and Hospitals of the American Medical Association utilizes three such subdivisions, defined respectively as major, minor, or for graduate training only.

A major teaching hospital is one, irrespective of whether it is university-owned or independent and under its own governing board, that is used extensively for the clinical instruction of medical school students. In fact, its educational role is far broader than this, but for our immediate purposes, the degree of involvement in student teaching is the important criterion. Conversely, a minor teaching hospital is used for only a limited amount of student instruction, for example, occasional demonstrations or clinics, or perhaps a single specialized clerkship.

In cities with one or more medical schools, relatively

loose affiliations may be developed with private hospitals whose staffs are made up to a considerable extent of men who also hold medical school appointments and participate in the programs of the major teaching hospitals. These physicians recognize the advantages, in terms of the quality of patient care, that can be derived from house staff programs and are, thus, willing to teach in the private hospitals as well in order to justify endeavors in graduate training.

In quantitative terms, the *Directory of Internships and Residencies,* published by the American Medical Association's Council on Medical Education and Hospitals in the Association's Journal, indicates the categorization of teaching affiliations as follows:

Type of teaching affiliation	Number of hospitals
Major	227
Minor	118
Graduate training only	44

Thus, of the almost 5700 short-term general hospitals, only 3.9 percent are classified as having major teaching affiliations; but since this group of institutions, as already noted, tends to include a good many hospitals with more than 300 beds, the total percentage of short-term general hospital beds used for teaching is relatively high.

For purposes of the present discussion, it seems appropriate to focus on the relationships between medical schools and major teaching hospitals. In thus limiting the scope of this paper, I in no way intend to suggest that so-called minor teaching affiliations are unimportant; they are, however, much less complex. It is in the relationship between the medical school and its major teaching hospital or hospitals that one finds the major share of the problems

ROBERT J. GLASER, M.D.

and challenges generating the crisis facing the contemporary hospital.

HISTORICAL PERSPECTIVE AND THE DEVELOPMENT OF MEDICAL EDUCATION

In considering the present-day relationships between medical schools and their teaching hospitals, one can gain valuable historical perspective by reviewing sequentially the development (a) of medical education in this country, and (b) of the teaching hospital. Medical schools and teaching hospitals are now closely related, but this interrelation is a rather recent phenomenon; the high quality that presently characterizes medical education in the United States is the result in part of the happy interactions between medical schools and their teaching hospitals.

The first medical schools as such came on the scene as part of clerical universities in Italy in the Middle Ages. The body of medical knowledge, however, remained extremely small for a good many centuries. Indeed, until the nineteenth century, anatomy was not only the predominant subject of instruction but almost the only one taught. Gradually there were added descriptions of certain clinical syndromes, some surgery, and a very moderate amount of therapy, most of it empirical and much of it not only useless but often harmful.

The first two medical schools in this country were established shortly before the American Revolution. In 1765, the College of Philadelphia initiated a program of medical teaching that was the forerunner of the University of Pennsylvania's Medical School, and three years later, a similar effort was initiated in New York as the King's College Medical School, the predecessor of the Columbia University College of Physicians and Surgeons. The Harvard Medical School was founded in Cambridge in

10

1783, the year that marked the close of the American Revolution.

Unfortunately, although the first attempts at medical education in this country arose within the framework of universities, medicine did not in fact become a university discipline for more than a hundred years. A number of the first medical schools bore the names of universities, but they were all essentially proprietary enterprises. Further, only a relatively small percentage of the physicians of the time actually obtained their education in the rudimentary institutions that then existed. It is said, for example, that in the early part of the nineteenth century, only 10 percent of the physicians of the time were graduates of the existing schools, and 80 percent had had no formal course work whatsoever. The primary route to medical practice was via an apprenticeship. In the days of the original colonies, as W. B. Wood points out in his Bampton Lectures at Columbia, the practice of medicine was often carried on by clergymen. [1] For most human ailments, there was so little known about treatment that the physician usually could offer only kindness to his patients, and sympathetic understanding, and often the clergymen of the time were the most effective dispensers of these supportive measures.

The development of proprietary medical schools throughout the nineteenth century went on at a great pace. During that span of 100 years, there were operating at one time or another in the United States more than 450 so-called medical schools. If one considers this figure in the light of the relatively small population of the time, and at the same time remembers that at present there are 85 or so schools operating and another 12 in the development state, one recognizes how very much simpler it must have been to establish and operate a medical school in that earlier period.

As already indicated, most of the medical schools were set up on a proprietary basis, often with profit as the major motive; education was a purely secondary consideration, if that. In many of the medical schools, the awarding of a degree was purely a formality, the sole prerequisite being receipt of a suitable fee by the proprietor(s). It is remarkable that there were produced, under the circumstances, so many worthy physicians. It is clear, as one reads historical accounts, that there were indeed a goodly number of physicians who, despite the handicap of limited knowledge, nonetheless ministered effectively and devotedly to their patients. They set a pattern of service to society that earned the physician an honored place in the fabric of the community.

In 1846, a group of dedicated physicians formed the American Medical Association in the hope of improving medical education and thus medical care in this country. Although progress was quite slow, the effort did go forward to upgrade standards.

In 1859, the first, graded medical curriculum was introduced at Northwestern University, and gradually there followed changes for the better in medical education. That the proprietary school influence persisted nonetheless is evidenced by the fact that as late as 1880 there were 11,800 medical students, a figure that rose to 27,650 in 1903; during this twenty-three year period, there was a 133 percent increase in the number of medical schools at a time when the country's population had only increased by 50 percent.

The organization of the Association of American Medical Colleges in 1890 constituted another step toward the achievement of high standards of medical education. In many respects, the founding of the Johns Hopkins University Medical School in 1893 was a major milestone, for there was created for the first time a truly university-oriented institution for graduate education. Under the remarkable and farsighted leadership of President Daniel Coit Gilman and Dr. William H. Welch, the standards of medical education were set at a level that even by today's standards was impressive.

It is not inappropriate to note that President Eliot of Harvard had a role in the development of Johns Hopkins, for he served as a consultant to the Hopkins Board and as an advisor to President Gilman. This point is well documented by Abraham Flexner in his excellent biography of Gilman. [2] Eliot, almost immediately upon the assumption of the presidency of Harvard in 1869, had concerned himself quite directly with the affairs of the medical school, but not with the overwhelming approval of the then senior faculty members. He recognized that the Harvard Medical School was not a part of the university in a real sense, and he took some steps to make it so. Some years ago, Dean George P. Berry recounted an interesting bit of history about the forces which brought about the integration of the Harvard Medical School into the university. Because this episode bears on the whole question of the development of medical education in this country and is not without its humorous side, I am going to take the liberty of quoting from Dr. Berry's account, as he presented it before the Association of American Medical Colleges in 1957.

Until 1869, the connection of the Medical School with Harvard College had been merely nominal, with the Governing Boards simply conferring the degrees voted by the Faculty of Medicine and confirming the professorial appointments made by them. The Faculty elected the Dean and otherwise conducted its affairs in an autonomous fashion. Then, in 1869, Charles Eliot became President of Harvard.

Mr. Eliot gave the first hint of what was coming when he took the chair at a meeting of the Faculty of Medicine — no

Harvard President had ever done so before. The crying need for a radical change from a proprietary to a university school and for the proper teaching of advancing science had caught his attention. A majority of the Professors in the Medical School were traditionally conservative, but a few allied themselves with the new President.

The champion of the conservatives was a surgeon of the Massachusetts General Hospital, distinguished in his day, Henry Jacob Bigelow. It was he who, at a later Faculty meeting, asked why so many changes were proposed when everything at the Medical School was quiet and prosperous. For a moment there was dead silence at the meeting. Then President Eliot replied, with the firm softness that characterized many of his utterances: "I can tell Dr. Bigelow the reason; we have a new President."

Dr. Bigelow objected to the higher requirements for entrance to the Medical School, advocated by the President, on the grounds that physicians and surgeons are born, not made, and that the inevitable reduction in numbers might exclude a genius in the art. He insisted that collateral sciences, which the medical student might or might not need, should not be confounded with the medical art, which he must have. He even denied that great medical discoveries are made in laboratories.

Finally, when Mr. Eliot and his adherents had carried the battle to the Harvard Corporation, Dr. Bigelow exclaimed: "Does the Corporation hold opinions on medical education? Who are the Corporation? Does Mr. Lowell know anything about medical education? Or the Reverend Putnam? Or Mr. Bowditch? Why, Mr. Crowninshield carries a horse chestnut in his pocket to keep off rheumatism! Is the new medical education to be best directed by a man who carries horse chestnuts in his pocket to cure rheumatism?"

The results of Mr. Eliot's battle are well known. The Medical School became an intimate and significant part of Harvard University. Within a year, Oliver Wendell Holmes, then a member of the Faculty of Medicine, wrote to a friend: "Our new President, Eliot, has turned the whole University over like a flapjack. There never was such a bouleversement as that in our Medical Faculty."

Mr. Eliot described the situation somewhat differently two years later when he wrote in his President's Report for 1871–1872: "It would be difficult to over-state the importance of the effort which this single school is making, with no support except the approval of the profession, to improve the system of medical instruction in the United States. The ignorance and general incompetency of the average graduate of American medical schools, at the time when he receives the degree which turns him loose upon the community, is something horrible to contemplate, considering the nature of a physician's functions and responsibilities." Mr. Eliot continued by emphasizing how much more devastating are the mistakes of a physician than are those of professionals in other walks of life. "The mistakes of an ignorant or stupid young physician or surgeon mean poisoning, maiming, and killing, or, at the best, they mean failure to save life and health which might have been saved, and to prevent suffering which might have been prevented . . . the Harvard Medical School has successfully begun a revolution in this system."

But to return to Mr. Crowninshield (of the Corporation) and his horse chestnut. He was asked if he did, indeed, carry a horse chestnut in his pocket to ward off rheumatism. He replied that he did carry a horse chestnut in his pocket. And did it work? Mr. Crowninshield thought it might be said that the horse chestnut was effective — in any event, the fact was that he had had no attacks of rheumatism since he had carried a horse chestnut in his pocket. Then, Mr. Crowninshield amplified his statement by expressing his amazement at the retroactive influence of the horse chestnut — the fact was, he said, he had had no attacks of rheumatism before he started carrying the horse chestnut! [3]

Harvard and President Eliot notwithstanding, however, the Johns Hopkins became the first medical school to require a college degree of its applicants, and although the leadership of the Hopkins group in defining stringent criteria for the admission of students was not immediately taken up by many other schools, most of which admitted students without even a high school diploma, it nonetheless ultimately had its effect. Even more important was the incorporation of the full-time principle in the basic science departments wherein men whose consuming interest was the education of medical students and the creation of new knowledge through the medium of research headed the several programs. It is a remarkable tribute to the founders of the Hopkins that the concept of full-time teachers has come to be a universally accepted keystone of modern medical education. Today, there are no medical schools that do not have a nucleus of full-time teachers on their medical faculties, and in most institutions full-time teachers now head and staff not only the basic science departments but the clinical departments as well, the latter pattern again having been established first at Johns Hopkins.

It is proper here to take note of the fact that teaching in the clinical departments of most medical schools is provided not only by full-time faculty members based in the teaching hospitals but also by able volunteer or part-time faculty members in private practice, men who contribute significantly to the over-all effectiveness of the education of medical students and of house officers.

In 1904, the Council on Medical Education of the American Medical Association was founded. That year, there were still 160 medical schools in the United States, 60 of them members of the Association of American Medical Colleges. That their standards of admission were still relatively low is demonstrated by the fact that on its founding in 1904, one of the council's first acts was to demand of its member schools that high school graduation be established as a minimal requirement for entry to medical school.

During the same period, the creation by a number of states of licensing boards had a role in raising standards. It became necessary, at least in some states, for those who wished to practice medicine to demonstrate in positive fashion their qualifications for the pursuit of their profession. In 1906, the American Medical Association, through its Council on Medical Education and Hospitals, attempted to grade medical schools. Three categories were established: A — acceptable, B — doubtful, and C — unacceptable. This program, representing as it did an important effort to achieve higher standards, was fraught with difficulties. Accusations of prejudice were directed on the part of the poorer schools toward the American Medical Association. It is not surprising that the loudest cries of protest often came from the proprietary enterprises. As I have already indicated, many of these schools were primarily operated for the enrichment of their proprietors, who had little or no concern for education per se. As one might have predicted, this abortive attempt at accreditation was not successful, but it is of interest to note in passing that the connotation of graded medical schools persisted for many years — even today, one occasionally hears from an uninformed layman that a given school is Grade A or B or C.

The recognition that drastic steps were in order led the Council on Medical Education of the American Medical Association to invite the Carnegie Corporation in 1908 to conduct an independent survey of the status of medical education in the United States. The Carnegie Corporation commissioned Mr. Abraham Flexner to make this survey, an assignment which can be properly described as Herculean, particularly in the first decade of this century when travel was far less comfortable and far more time-consuming than it is today. Further, because of the wretched state of medical education in general, the mission did not promise to be very gratifying. Indeed, the magnitude of the task facing Flexner was somewhat similar to that which confronted Hercules when he undertook to

clean the Augean stables. Mr. Flexner recognized the
breadth of this assignment and the many unpleasant
aspects characterizing it. Nonetheless, with unfailing interest and prodigious energy, he undertook to visit all the
medical schools in the United States, and in his monu-
mental "Bulletin No. 4," published in 1910 by the Carnegie
Corporation he presented his findings, which documented
the deplorable state that characterized the great majority
of medical schools. [4] In a few schools, as had been the
case decades earlier, the organization was little more than
a paper one, and a student had only to register and pay the
requisite tuition to obtain the degree of Doctor of Medicine. In many, the facilities were inadequate, formal
courses few, and the approach purely didactic.

The lack of appropriate medical school–teaching hospital relationships was a common and striking finding. For
example, when Flexner visited the Harvard Medical School
in 1909, he made the following observations on this point:

Abundant clinical material is available at the Massachusetts
General Hospital, the City Hospital, and elsewhere. But serious restrictions are felt in two directions: (1) while the university is free to secure laboratory men wherever it chooses,
it is practically bound to make clinical appointments by seniority, in accordance with the custom prevailing in the hospital
which it uses, or to leave its professor without a hospital clinic.
In general, it follows that the heir to the hospital service is
heir to the university chair. In consequence, there is a notice-
able lack of sympathy between the laboratory and the clinical
men. They do not represent the same ideals. There is no question but that an institution of this rank ought to work in the
most intimate cooperation with a hospital; and that, if such were
the case, the same principles would obtain in selecting clinical
teachers as prevail elsewhere in the university. (2) The extent
to which hospital material can be utilized is also limited,
though less in surgery than in medicine. The teaching is in
the main of the demonstrative character. [5]

Many of the changes that have brought medical education to its present high state occurred after publication of the Flexner Report in 1910; it was from that date that there was a steady disappearance from the scene of the diploma mills and the hopelessly inferior schools, and concomitantly the upgrading of standards at the remaining schools as they began to identify in fact as well as in name with universities. More and more full-time faculty members were appointed, both in the basic sciences and the clinical departments, and the pursuit of research began to be a more prominent part of the medical school program.

The great private foundations played an immense role in upgrading medical education. The Rockefeller Foundation, both directly and through its General Education Board, made a number of significant grants which created some of the schools that became leaders in medical education. Among these, in addition to the Hopkins, were the Washington University School of Medicine in St. Louis, and somewhat later, the University of Rochester School of Medicine. The Rockefeller Foundation and the Commonwealth Fund, by supporting research activity and making possible the appointment of outstanding scientists on medical faculties, paved the way for the subsequent developments which have contributed so much to our understanding of medical problems.

GROWTH OF RESEARCH IN MEDICINE

During World War II, it became clearly demonstrated that major efforts in the field of scientific research and development were identified with results which had great import for the population as a whole. In the case of the Manhattan Project, which resulted in the atomic bomb, the development had a very alarming potential, but it is well to remember that the peaceful uses of atomic energy also

ROBERT J. GLASER, M.D.

have great possibilities for good, both in medicine and in industry. In medicine per se, the development of penicillin constituted an illustration of how research can bring great and important practical results. Penicillin was discovered by Fleming in 1929 but it remained a scientific curiosity for a number of years. In 1941, as a result of studies by Florey and others, it became clear that this antimicrobial substance had great potential for the treatment of life-threatening infections, and a major effort was mounted to produce it in significant quantities.

I well remember the exciting days when penicillin was introduced into clinical medicine. As a house officer, I had the opportunity of participating in a nationwide project designed to evaluate penicillin in the treatment of bacterial endocarditis, a disease that hitherto had been almost universally fatal. The drug was in such short supply and was so valuable that we kept it locked in a vault and distributed it in what today would seem to be tiny quantities and only after extremely critical evaluation of each patient's problem. Within the space of several years, by virtue of the initiation of a crash program that brought to bear the talents and resources of many scientists and of industry, particularly the fermentation industry, penicillin became plentiful, and it was not long thereafter before the vials in which the drug was packaged were more expensive than the drug itself. The subsequent development of a number of other life-saving antimicrobial agents demonstrated in dramatic fashion how research could change the whole fabric of medicine. As a result, the people of this country, through their elected representatives, made it clear that they favored research support on a large scale, and in the past fifteen to twenty years, support of biomedical research by the federal government has grown to immense proportions. In the current fiscal year, for example, the National

Institutes of Health alone are budgeting over a billion dollars for biomedical research.

I have dwelt on this growth of research as part of my historical survey of the development of medical education because it has been the single factor that has had the most profound effect on medical schools in the past quarter of a century.

The availability of research funds on a large basis made possible the expansion of faculties in many medical schools where such expansion had not previously been possible. Medical schools, other than those proprietary enterprises which existed chiefly on paper, have never been adequately financed. The financial problems today, though different, are certainly not less significant than they were twenty years ago. Indeed, in many ways they are much more severe. Nonetheless, the addition to faculties of able grant-supported scientists, many of whom not only pursued imaginative investigative programs but at the same time contributed to teaching and to patient care, improved medical education significantly.

To accommodate the great research effort, there have been major additions to the physical facilities of medical schools, and their budgets have mushroomed. The burgeoning of knowledge has in turn made the teaching hospital the scene of tremendous growth and change. Whereas prior to World War II much of the research that went on took place in the basic science departments, and only a relatively small amount of research was carried on by clinical departments, in the past decade or two immense research activity has been undertaken by clinical departments. Indeed, in more than a few medical schools in 1965, a department of medicine or a department of surgery may number as many full-time members as the entire faculty of the same school did twenty-five years ago.

ROBERT J. GLASER, M.D.

Clearly this magnitude of change in program has had a significant impact on the teaching hospital and its medical school.

THE TEACHING HOSPITAL

Let us turn now to a brief history of the development of the teaching hospital in America. Again, because of the rather unsophisticated and rather didactic character of medicine until the modern era, there was remarkably little attention paid to hospital facilities by those concerned with medical education until the turn of this century. Students saw little or nothing of patients and were expected to gain clinical experience only after they received the M.D. degree. It is true that a number of the earliest hospitals in this country were considered to be available for the teaching of students and physicians, even though this aspect of the hospital program was minimal. For example, the Pennsylvania Hospital, founded in 1751, in large part through the efforts of Benjamin Franklin, was the first hospital in this country that conformed to our present concept of an acute general hospital. In rules adopted in 1772, provision was made for the admission of apprentices or students of medicine, and teaching of a sort, therefore, did go on within the walls of that institution almost from its founding.

Similarly, when the effort to establish the Massachusetts General Hospital was being pursued, two of its founders, Dr. John Collins Warren and Dr. James Jackson, prepared a letter setting forth their views on the role of the teaching hospital in medical education, as follows:

The means of medical education in New England are at present very limited, and totally inadequate to so important a purpose. . . . Those who are educated in New England have so few opportunities of attending to the practice of physic,

22

that they find it impossible to learn some of the most important elements of the science of medicine, until after they have undertaken for themselves the care of the health and lives of their fellow-citizens. This care they undertake with very little knowledge, except that acquired from books. . . . With such deficiencies in medical education, it is needless to show to what evils the community is exposed. . . . A hospital is an institution absolutely essential to a medical school, and one which would afford relief and comfort to thousands of the sick and miserable. On what other objects can the superfluities of the rich be so well bestowed? [6]

J. E. Garland, in his brief history of the Massachusetts General Hospital, pays tribute to the Jackson-Warren letter, described as "the cornerstone of the Hospital." It brought forth an "immediate and enthusiastic" response and within six months led to the granting of a charter for the hospital. The legislative committee of the Massachusetts General Court, in its report recommending approval of the charter, concluded with an important observation, acknowledging that committee's appreciation of the teaching function of the hospital: "The location of the proposed Hospital is intended to be such as will accommodate students in the metropolis and at the University in Cambridge, and the skill thus acquired, by the increased means of instruction, will be gradually and constantly diffused through every section of the Commonwealth." [7] But despite the vision and wisdom of Drs. Jackson and Warren, and the interest of the legislators of the time, clinical teaching, at least in the undergraduate curriculum, remained limited, and medical schools in general paid little attention to the question of a teaching hospital affiliation.

Two factors ultimately led to an increased role for the teaching hospital. One was the development of the forerunners of internship and residency, which have become such a key part of modern medical education. As early as

1800, it was recognized that clinical experience was an important requisite for the physician, and in New York at the Bellevue Hospital, among other institutions, there developed the forerunner of the modern house officership. Around 1900, the so-called graduate programs began to be emphasized on a major scale. Again, it was the Johns Hopkins group which had a key role in this regard. Sir William Osler and William S. Halsted, respectively the first Professors of Medicine and of Surgery at the Hopkins, were impressed with what they had seen in the German clinics, where a young physician spent a number of years under his chief, gaining clinical experience. They adopted this general approach in Baltimore, and from there it spread broadly.

The second factor leading to increased use of the teaching hospital, in which Osler also had a key role, came as the result of the creation of what are now called clinical clerkships. By introducing medical students to the patient at his bedside, Osler and his confreres made the teaching hospital an integral part of the medical school. The clinical laboratories were comparable in their role in the third and fourth years of medicine to the basic science laboratories in the first two years. The Johns Hopkins Hospital had been built contiguous to the medical school and from the outset was designed to support teaching, both at the undergraduate and graduate levels.

The Hopkins example was copied widely, and as medical students and house officers became directly involved, under appropriate supervision, in patient care, the teaching hospital assumed a more and more significant role in medical education. In the period since 1900, there has been actually much greater expansion, in terms of scope of programs, within the teaching hospitals than there has been within the basic sciences. This is not to suggest that the basic sciences have not themselves been the scene of tremendous expansion. The basic sciences, after all, form the foundation of all medicine. On the other hand, as I have already noted earlier, the growth of full-time clinical departments and of research programs within those departments has been percentage-wise greater than the growth of the basic science departments, and there has resulted an enormous increase in the educational and research role or the teaching hospital.

THE MEDICAL CENTER

As medical education became more and more identified as a joint venture between the medical school and the teaching hospital, there inevitably evolved what today we call the medical center. Again, it is of historical interest to recognize that the concept of placing a medical school and a hospital contiguous one to the other was not always looked on favorably. In this connection, it is well worth remembering that, when the faculty of the Harvard Medical School planned to move from Cambridge to Boston in order to be closer to clinical facilities, an inquiry was directed by the Medical School Faculty to the Trustees of the Massachusetts General Hospital asking whether or not that body would be interested in having the Medical School built adjacent to the MGH. The trustees replied without much delay that they did not see any advantage to accrue from this suggestion and indeed saw some distinct disadvantages. [8] As things turned out, the MGH fortunately did remain an integral part of the whole Harvard medical teaching scene, but it is entirely within the realm of possibility that such might not have been the case.

I have already pointed out that the Johns Hopkins Hospital was built adjacent to the Hopkins Medical School in order to support teaching in an effective way. In a sense, this was the first university medical center in the country, and William H. Welch, who was a key figure in charting the course of the Hopkins as its first dean, spoke often of the importance of a close and meaningful association between medical school and hospital. He perceived clearly the role of the teaching hospital, both in terms of education and in the creation of new knowledge, while concomitantly it provided the locus for exemplary patient care. He was joined by Flexner in forwarding the concept that there should be a close union between medical schools and hospitals.

In 1912, Welch spoke at the forty-third anniversary of the Presbyterian Hospital in New York and expressed the hope that the hospital and the College of Physicians and Surgeons of Columbia University would ultimately come into association side by side. [9] It was exactly twenty years later that the two institutions were united into a single physical complex, and as Houston Merritt noted recently, the Columbia-Presbyterian Medical Center was the first to be so titled. [10]

The Flexner Report influenced the development of other great university medical centers in this country, for example, the Cornell Medical College–New York Hospital, the Yale Medical School–New Haven Hospital, the Washington University Medical School–Barnes Hospital, and the Western Reserve University Medical School–Lakeside Hospital.

Until World War II, the union between medical schools and hospitals grew in size and complexity, but they were still relatively simple entities, at least by today's standards. Full-time faculties were small; the internship and residency programs, modest; postdoctoral fellowship programs were few in numbers; and research was still limited.

After World War II, by virtue of the changes that have

already been described, the modern university medical center came into being. It is a far more complex organization than most people realize. Traditionally, the program of the medical school and its teaching hospital has been a threefold one — education, research, and patient care, and this is still the case. On the other hand, one need only look at any one of these areas to realize how the scope of each one has broadened. Just as the full-time staffs of clinical departments have increased, so has the research effort going forward within these departments been expanded, so that it is not uncommon for a single major clinical department to have a research budget of well over a million dollars annually. The research budget of the Massachusetts General Hospital alone, now of the order of ten million dollars, is greater than the entire research budget of a good many university medical centers in the country.

NEWER DEVELOPMENTS — EXPECTATIONS AND PROBLEMS

The patient care programs and teaching at the undergraduate and particularly at the graduate level have grown apace. As new knowledge comes on the scene at an ever-increasing rate, indeed exponentially, there are new opportunities in patient care, and concomitantly in teaching and research. Whole new fields within clinical medicine have developed in direct relationship to new knowledge or more thorough understanding of existing knowledge. The new knowledge in genetics and immunology, for example, has had profound effects on the scope of the patient care and educational programs in our teaching hospitals. Some of the benefits that have accrued to patients are well known, while others are not so well appreciated. Consider, for purposes of illustration, the entity known as phenylketonuria.

When I was a third-year medical student in the out-

27

patient department of the Massachusetts General a bit over twenty years ago, one of my classmates, who had been a biochemist before entering medical school, astounded one and all when he performed a simple laboratory test and recognized that the result pointed to the diagnosis of phenylketonuria. This disease, though not common, is not rare and may cause profound mental retardation. There are significant numbers of patients in our mental institutions, doomed to a custodial existence, because of this inborn metabolic error. In 1942, its recognition constituted only evidence of diagnostic erudition — nothing could be done for the unfortunate patient.

Consider then the fruits of the laboratory investigation of this syndrome: in brief, the inability of certain patients to convert the amino acid tryptophane to tyrosine. These patients lack an enzyme, phenylalanine hydroxylase, which catalyzes the conversion. Further, we have a relatively simple method by which newborns may be screened for this disorder. If the correct diagnosis is made promptly after birth, modification of the diet normally given infants can prevent mental retardation. In short, the disease is now preventable.

Current literature contains reference to increasing numbers of other diseases that represent inborn errors of metabolism, and in some instances, research findings have resulted in effective methods of prevention or treatment. The point is that our widening knowledge constantly provides new opportunities to prevent or treat disease or at least to alleviate suffering.

It is in the teaching hospitals that the frontiers of clinical medicine lie. There is no single area of the teaching hospitals that is not affected by the exciting advances everywhere about us in medicine and the sciences basic to medicine. Consequently, there is a never-ending demand on these institutions for personnel, space, and equipment, and all of these spell "money."

In some ways, the situation is not unlike that which is familiar to us in the fable of the Sorcerer's Apprentice. The process of producing new knowledge has been turned on and it can't be turned off. Whereas in the fable, there was reason to stop the flow of water before all was washed away before it, when the product is new knowledge resulting in continuing benefits to our fellows, there is no thought of turning off the flow — rather, there is concern about how best to harness the fortuitous flood in order to exploit it maximally.

Even if we in medicine did not wish to do so, we would have no choice. For in this same period since the end of World War II, there has occurred a dramatic change in the expectations of the public in respect to medical care. To a considerable degree, these changing expectations reflect the public's recognition of the contributions of research to better understanding of the problems of disease and their control.

The advent of the antibiotics, of heart surgery, and more recently of transplantation, all widely publicized, has emphasized in dramatic fashion the enhanced potential of medical care for the public good. Patients now look to quality health care as a right rather than as a privilege, and the demands on the great urban teaching hospitals, in the sphere of patient care, are growing daily. One need only examine one area in an institution like the Massachusetts General Hospital, namely, the emergency ward, to realize how much greater a role, in the day-to-day care of patients, the urban teaching hospital is playing. In this institution and in others like it, probably 50 percent of the patients who come to the emergency ward do not have life-threatening illness. Rather, they recognize that quality medical care is available here day and night. They know that a superior staff of intern and resident physicians and excellent laboratories, all functioning on a twenty-four hour basis, are available to meet their needs, and understandably they turn to this hospital when illness strikes. The patient also comes to the emergency ward by referral of his private physician or because he is unable to reach him in time of need.

The fact that in many urban areas, and especially in less affluent ones, the number of physicians is decreasing, tends to increase the dependence of the populace in such areas on the teaching hospital, not only for consultation and major problems, as was formerly the case, but also for less serious medical needs.

As Dr. Knowles has pointed out, the community looks to the teaching hospital to fulfill a broader role than it did a few decades ago; [11] concomitantly, the teaching hospital must perforce look at the community and at its role differently than it did in days gone by. In this context, let me cite a paragraph from an important publication which made its appearance in 1953:

The university teaching hospital must guard its staff and faculty members from unduly large service responsibilities. As the number of patients increases, the faculty must be expanded or its members will have insufficient time for research and for the instruction of students. This principle was clearly understood by physicians interested in medical education and was put into effect in many instances when funds became available early in the century for the construction of university-owned hospitals. In recent years, such institutions have at times deprecatingly been called "ivory towers" because they did not attempt to serve all or a large part of the immediate needs of the community. Actually, these institutions have been leaders of progress in medical knowledge in the study of diseases. They developed investigation bringing the basic sciences to bear directly on the problems of illness. The residency system of training which has produced the faculties of our medical schools was born and has flourished in such "ivory towers." [12]

The foregoing paragraph states a principle that is still an important one, namely, that if the teaching hospital staff is to discharge its obligations in the areas of creating new knowledge and of educating tomorrow's physicians, it cannot be overburdened with patient care. On the other hand, the day is probably passed when a great teaching hospital can continue to operate on the basis of accepting only those patients who "are good teaching material," to the exclusion of others. The teaching hospital's obligation to the community precludes such a policy.

The teaching hospital cannot be all things to all men. It cannot provide all the medical care that is to be provided in a large urban area. On the other hand, it must recognize its responsibility to the community, particularly in respect to the development of models of quality patient care that can subsequently be adopted in other institutions that do not have as their primary function, or even as one of their functions, the teaching of medical students and house officers. This role is one of the responsibilities of leadership that the teaching hospitals must continue to accept.

As the teaching hospital's patient care programs continue to grow and become more rather than less diversified, and as the teaching hospital becomes more involved on the one hand with the translation of new knowledge into practical application and on the other in serving, if you will, as the family doctor for segments of the population, its additional needs, both in terms of personnel and facilities, must be met. The faculty members who make up the hospital's professional personnel will be recruited primarily by the medical school, but by virtue of the fact that they will be using the hospital's facilities, there will have to be the closest cooperation between the two bodies. Where the university owns the hospital and one board governs both enterprises, there is essentially no problem. On the other hand, where hospital and medical school are governed and administered separately, as is true in the Harvard system and in a good many others, especially in the private university medical centers, an effective liaison mechanism between the governing boards is needed. The proper allocation of costs is itself a very major problem; few expenses directly related to teaching and research should be charged to the patient.

Earlier I pointed out that medical schools have been underfinanced almost from the beginning. The diploma mills, of course, had no problem in this regard, but once institutions whose objectives were genuinely directed toward good education came on the scene, the financial pinch began to be felt. In earlier years when there was little technology involved, costs in this respect were minimal. And as essentially all teaching was provided on a volunteer basis, faculty salaries were inconsequential.

As full-time faculties were appointed, and as the technical sophistication of medicine advanced, costs began to mount, and by now they are of impressive magnitude. I earlier noted that it is not uncommon for several departments within a medical school each to have a budget of well over a million dollars; of the total budget, however, the amount derived from research grants is usually large, often of the order of 50 to 60 percent or even 75 percent.

We must not lose sight of the fact that research grants have been the means by which able teachers and clinicians have been brought into the medical school and its teaching hospitals. There has thus been added an able complement of physicians and basic scientists who have made notable contributions to the educational and patient care programs of the teaching hospitals as they carry out their research. Yet the terms of most research grants understandably limit the time that investigators can devote to nonresearch pursuits. Hence, no matter how large the research budget, the need for a respectable "hard money base," to be used for salaries of professional staff, is not obviated. Indeed, if appropriate balance is to be maintained, this budgetary component should increase in some reasonable proportion with the research budget. That this has not been the case in most of our medical schools and certainly in the clinical departments in the teaching hospitals is painfully obvious.

And, sad to relate, there is a further complication, namely, the indirect expenses chargeable to research — the provision of the costs of mundane items such as heat, light, janitor service, and maintenance. That there are indirect expenses is recognized by granting agencies and most of them include a budgetary item so identified. But the amounts allocated to meet these costs are frequently inadequate, and the institutions — either the schools or the hospitals — must use their own internal funds to make up the difference. The pursuit of research, a *sine qua non* in a program of excellence, has therefore added a financial burden of major proportion. The relative size of the teaching hospital research program, the limited amounts of unrestricted income available from endowments, and the lack of tuition income has in many instances contributed to the hospital's current crisis. I want to emphasize the fact that the problems in this area are serious and will continue to be, for we can expect little respite from new capital needs and additions to the operating budgets of our hospitals. We must always keep in mind the fact that the new financial demands reflect only in part the inflationary spiral of the times as the cost of living rises; they also are the price of advancing knowledge and of applying for the benefit of our patients the fruits of laboratory research.

There is, of course, a tremendous economic dividend directly related to the advances being made in the teaching hospital, if you will, a dividend resulting from our investment in research. Unfortunately, the hospitals can at best benefit only indirectly from the dividend. I refer, of course, to the gigantic saving represented by decreased human suffering and lessened incapacitation, and the resultant immense gain in human productivity attributable to advances in the prevention and treatment of disease.

Consider only the cost of custodial care of one mentally retarded human being, care which by and large leaves much to be desired. Such an unfortunate patient requires institutional care for his entire lifetime, and this period may be sixty or seventy years in duration. For one such patient, assuming a total daily maintenance cost of only five dollars, the cost for a sixty-year period would be over $100,000. Further, remember that this same individual, were he not handicapped and instead able to lead a productive life, could be expected to contribute positively to society. Then replicate this single example thousands of times and you will readily see what I mean by the dividend of our investment in health.

I would suggest that this consideration should enter into all examinations of the high cost of medical care, for it provides a sound basis for public support of medical schools and their teaching hospitals, the vehicles by which medicine advances.

One other factor contributes to the cost of care in teaching hospitals. Their beds are occupied in high proportion by patients with complicated and life-threatening disease problems, and the care of these patients is inevitably costly.

Yet it is precisely this kind of care that the teaching hospitals can provide best. They are a unique resource with a unique role. They complement the many fine nonteaching hospitals in a given region, and together these institutions, through the devoted services of their physicians, nurses, and other personnel, assure quality health care for our citizens.

In the years ahead, it seems reasonable to suggest that all the costs of medical care per se should be met by the patient, either directly or via insurance carriers and governmental agencies. At the same time, the costs of education and research will have to be met by the institutions — the medical schools and the teaching hospitals. I believe we can safely assume that much of the cost of research, including the major endeavors in clinical research represented by the relatively new categorical and noncategorical centers, can be funded from extramural sources, chiefly the National Institutes of Health. Is there any mechanism by which funds may be obtained to support the other very major item in the teaching hospital budget, the salaries of the full-time professional staff? I believe there is.

Those who elect full-time careers should be paid attractive salaries, in return for which they can be expected to devote appropriate portions of their time to patient care, teaching, and research. Obviously one cannot arbitrarily define the amount of time that faculty members should devote to each of these activities. It is clear, however, that within the limits of the patient care program undertaken by the teaching hospital, members of the faculty must be willing to meet the resultant clinical obligations.

In turn the professional fees for patient care, which are becoming available in steadily increasing amounts by virtue of the growth of insurance plans, should be used for the support of the full-time group as a whole rather than accrue in disproportionate amounts to relatively few of its members. I believe the time has come for medical schools, their parent universities, and their affiliated teaching hospitals to recognize that some form of strict full-time organization is the best means of achieving long-term financial stability. This is neither the time nor the place to enter into a detailed discussion of the design of a strict full-time system. The principles are simple: the system must be one in which there is neither exploitation of faculty members by the institutions nor of the institution by the faculty members. The success of the strict full-time system and its practicality is attested to in a number of outstanding university medical centers; both privately and publicly supported.

In this connection, I should like to make one other point. The development of teaching hospitals as we know them today would not have been possible without internship and residency programs; when properly constituted, these programs are admirable instruments that combine continuing graduate education with quality service.

The essentiality of the house staff to the achievement of the teaching hospital's goals needs no supporting brief here. What must be emphasized is the necessity of paying adequate salaries, adequate in terms of the professional qualifications to our house officers.

Here again, the patient should not be expected to bear this burden entirely. In part, the salaries of the house staff are a proper charge to patients in recognition of the services provided. On the other hand, that portion of house officer time which is devoted to teaching — and a good bit is — and to the young physician's own continuing education should be funded by other means.

Professional fees, available via insurance, represent a sound means of meeting this problem. Particularly should Blue Shield payments be recovered for care rendered by house officers. It is indeed paradoxical that a young physician, just out of his internship and in private practice, can receive Blue Shield payments for care of patients without any issue whatsoever being made. Yet in many states, the professional services of advanced residents, with much more experience and mature clinical judgment, are not reimbursable by Blue Shield. Here is a place where organized medicine, through its responsibility for setting Blue Shield policy, can make a great contribution to medical education, the teaching hospital, and the future members of our profession.

These are times of vast change in politics, in science, in medicine, in all facets of society, here and all over the world. The relationships between medical schools and teaching hospitals and between teaching hospitals and society are intimately affected in the process. Change is rarely easy, particularly when it involves complex entities. But change we must, even though, as Steinbeck reminds us, "it is in the nature of man — to protest change, particularly change for the better." [13] And long before Steinbeck, Machiavelli wrote, "It must be considered that there is nothing more difficult to carry out, nor more doubtful of success, nor more dangerous to handle, than to initiate a new order of things." [14]

We face, if not a new order of things, at least a rapidly changing order, and the crisis facing the contemporary hospital is part of it. The crisis carries with it a challenge; the challenge is an exciting one, for it offers medicine the opportunity to make the lives of our citizens freer from disease and suffering than ever was possible before. It is mandatory, therefore, that we support our medical schools and teaching hospitals in a manner which will allow them to embellish their proud records of achievement and their contribution to society.

SURGERY IN A
TIME OF CHANGE

Paul S. Russell, M.D.

INSTITUTIONS like the Massachusetts General Hospital
face issues of varying importance almost every day. The
most problematic are those related to the difficulties of
people accepting change. Wilfred Trotter, that intrepid
British surgeon, wrote in 1932, "The mind delights in a
static environment, and if there is any change to be itself
the source. Change from without, interfering as it must
with the sovereignty of the individual, seems in its very
essence to be repulsive and an object of fear." [1]

Nevertheless, difficult as change may be, surgery has
been deeply involved as an active contributor to the great
sweep of change which is continually working through our
society in all its aspects, seemingly with steadily greater
rapidity. Even glimpses of the surgeon at work give some
idea of the great changes which have been wrought in his
activities. (See Figures 1A–D.)

No matter how complicated the procedure, it is important to remember that surgical treatment is directed to the
single patient and represents an especially impressive example of the concern we all have in Western society for
the welfare of the individual. Nowadays this individual
patient has at his disposal a galaxy of supporting special

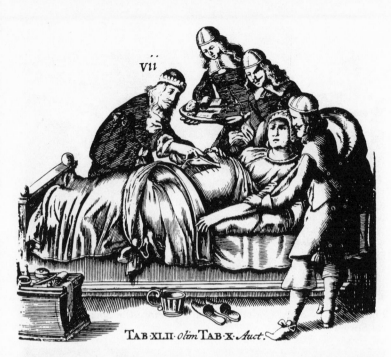

Figure 1(A). A Caesarean section as portrayed by Scultetus in his "Armamentarium Chirurgicum" in about 1600.

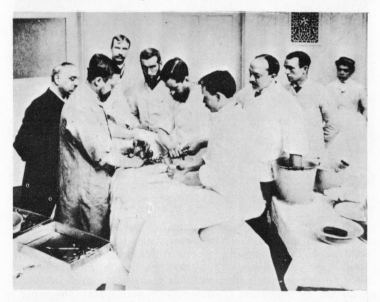

Figure 1(B). J. Collins Warren, assisted by S. Jason Mixter, performing the first operation in the Bradlee surgical amphitheater in 1889.

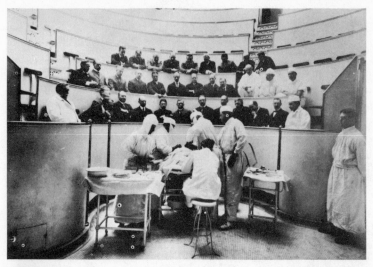

Figure 1(C). E. A. Codman operating before the Society of Clinical Surgery in 1908.

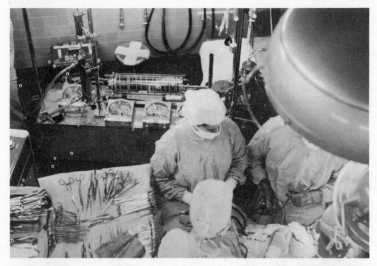

Figure 1(D). An open-heart operation at the Massachusetts General Hospital in 1965. It is apparent that the complexity of the operation itself has steadily increased, particularly in relatively recent times. Anesthesia and antisepsis had been introduced by 1889. An extension of antisepsis to early asepsis occurred by 1908, exemplified by the advent of rubber gloves and masks. The importance of teamwork and the reliance on instrumentation are apparent in the most recent photograph.

talents in the teaching hospital that would have been undreamed of at the time of this hospital's founding. Partly for this reason, surgical activities have been more and more confined to hospitals in the last fifty years. About 70 percent of patients admitted to most large, central hospitals such as the MGH undergo some form of surgical procedure in the operating room when they are there. In 1850 some 330 operations were performed in the single operating theater of the Massachusetts General Hospital at a time when about 135 patients of all sorts could be received at once. In those days, all were "ward" or charity patients, operations on private patients being commonly conducted at home. Last year, 17,061 operations were performed in the MGH's three operating suites, and the hospital has grown to a capacity of 1050 beds. At present, about 66 percent of our patients are in the private category.

THE NATURE OF SURGERY

How can surgery be defined, and what are some of its distinctive features? Clearly, the surgical method deals with localized processes or those in which action concentrated on a local area of the body will be helpful. The care of a wound or the removal of a foreign body are time-honored surgical assignments. As the history of medicine has unfolded, however, the surgical method has shown its usefulness in virtually every type of disease. Who would have supposed, for example, that the removal of a tiny tumor of a parathyroid gland from an obscure place deep in the neck, would prove to give dramatic relief from a generalized metabolic disease, sometimes manifested by severe crippling bony deformities and urinary stones? There can thus be no dispute as to the absolute necessity for the surgeon to be broadly educated in medicine, although much controversy has turned on this question in

the past, and I will return to it again. Celsus, the Roman
sage of the first Christian century, was ahead of his time
when he wrote, "The third part of the Art of Medicine is
that which cures by the hand, as I have already said, and
indeed it is common knowledge. It does not omit medica-
ments and regulated diets but does most by hand. The
effects of this treatment are more obvious than any other
kind." [2]

Celsus' broad approach to surgery has not been shared
generally, however, and many surgeons still have the repu-
tation of tending to concentrate not just on an individual
patient but exclusively on a certain localized portion of
him. Anyone who refers to "that gall bladder in Room 4"
is a distressing victim of this malady. This dangerous and
stultifying view springs from a preoccupation with tech-
nique. It is less common now than it was three or four
decades ago. Renewed emphasis on and understanding of
a broader view of man will become all the more imperative
as the complexity of surgical decisions increases. Cardinal
Newman's words elevate the problem to a grander scale
but suggest what I mean here:

Let us take, for example, man himself as our object of con-
templation; then at once we shall find we can view him in a
variety of relations; and according to those relations are the
sciences of which he is the subject matter, and according to
our acquaintance with them is our possession of a true knowledge of him. We may view him in relation to the material
elements of his body, or to his mental constitution, or to his
household and family, or to the community in which he lives,
or to the Being who made him; and in consequence we treat
him respectively as physiologists, or as moral philosophers, or
as writers of economics, or of politics, or as theologians. . . .
On the other hand, according as we are only physiologists, or
only politicians, or only moralists, so is our idea of man more
or less unreal. [3]

Thus not only must the surgeon, who carries responsibility for major intervention in the life of his patient, be prepared with knowledge of the details of the techniques to be applied locally, by appropriate familiarity and experience with them, but also he must be capable of taking full charge of his patient and of understanding the wider implications of his surgical acts. This is not to say that the surgeon of the future will become a contemplative philosopher since he will always have to be ready for the unexpected and be capable of speedy decisions even without all the information he might wish to have. ·Sir Heneage Ogilvie may have overdrawn the difference between medicine and surgery when he wrote,

A surgeon conducting a difficult case is like the skipper of an ocean-going yacht. He knows the port he must make but he cannot foresee the course of the journey. . . . The physician's task is more comparable to that of the golfer. . . . If he judges the direction and the wind right, estimates each lie correctly, finds the right club for each shot and uses it skillfully, he will get an eagle or a birdie. If he makes a mistake he will make a poor score, but will get there in the end. The ground will not split beneath his feet, the game will not change suddenly from golf to bull fighting. [4]

STRUCTURE, SCIENCE, AND SETTING OF SURGERY

What of some of the more significant changes that can be identified now in regard to surgery in the teaching hospital? I shall address myself especially to three of these: they are *structure, science,* and *setting,* that is, the organizational structure of surgery and its specialties, the development of science in surgery, and the imminent changes in the setting in which surgery is taught in the teaching hospitals. All these things are changing simultaneously and to some extent interdependently. Only the last one is of very recent origin.

It is generally assumed that the necessity for concentration of a high degree of skill in the case of a craftsman, or of imagination and inventiveness in the case of a scientist, upon a confined region of specialization comes from the pressing demands of his special area. These demands may, in certain instances, have to do with the scope of the intellectual problems concerned or the high level of special skill required. Specialties can, however, be determined on quite different grounds, grounds which depend more on the flow of work to be done rather on its difficulty. Obviously the latter type of specialty not only lacks intellectual stimulation but is especially vulnerable to elimination or transformation by virtue of advances or changes beyond its control. This kind of specialization tends to be undesirable in a teaching hospital for a number of reasons, the most important of which is that it sets a poor example for younger colleagues, as I will discuss later.

Structure. / We can think of the surgical specialty structure in an arboreal form. (Figure 2). One misleading implication in Figure 2 is that these various special areas were understood, at the time, to be related to one another or necessarily tied together. Actually, each tended to be practiced by a separate guild, and principles common to all were not generally recognized.

Recently a great burgeoning of specialization has taken place in surgery as in many other fields. More than ever, however, it is now of great importance that the supporting trunk of general surgery be a sturdy one (Figure 3). If general surgery is serving its purpose it should embody most of the concepts and techniques which are common to

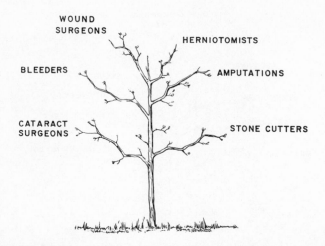

WOUND
SURGEONS

HERNIOTOMISTS

BLEEDERS

AMPUTATIONS

CATARACT
SURGEONS

STONE CUTTERS

Figure 2. A diagrammatic view of the "specialties" of surgery which might have been detected in about the sixteenth century. There was little understanding at the time of the unity of surgery now recognized to be important.

all the specialties. In this sense it is basic to the specialties and is their progenitor. The principles of wound management, of the metabolic shifts associated with injury and the management of infection, are examples of the most fundamental and durable of these. Experience in general surgery must, therefore, be an important and integrated portion of the development of all surgeons. This has been recognized by the various specialty boards which have assumed the duty of establishing desirable standards in the subdivisions of surgery, but coordination between them is still sadly lacking and often results in too parochial a view by each group. Proper coordination could lead to a well-planned course up the trunk of general surgery to a selected branch for the individual who chooses to devote himself to a specialty.

45

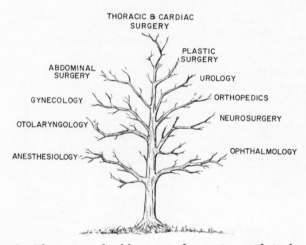

Figure 3. The present healthy surgical organism with its burgeoning specialties.

It is interesting to me that some of the most actively progressing areas of medicine and surgery alike now depend heavily upon a collaborative approach in which people of different clinical backgrounds are involved. Clinical cardiology is a good example. The exclusive approach, particularly typical of guilds with a financial vested interest, which results in protective fences about areas, perhaps has some advantages in maintaining standards of performance in the early history of a specialty but must not be allowed to crystallize specialties in a certain posture, particularly in a teaching hospital. The same warning is often voiced concerning university departments. Specialties should be free to draw back into the stem of general surgery, without the restraint of vested interests, where they will give way to new growing tips or branches from time to time. For example, some think that pulmonary surgery has now run its proper course as a specialty and should be reabsorbed into general surgery. In summary, the benefits of specialism are undeniable, but its hazards to progress and to the free exchange of ideas in teaching must be guarded against.

The Science of Surgery. What of the impact of biological science on the practical art of surgery, on the postgraduate teaching of surgery, and on the organization of surgical departments. Unquestionably, surgeons have opened many new avenues of progress as they probe into previously obscure regions of the body and draw the attention of others to previously unappreciated aspects of disease. The whole recent development of peripheral arterial recon- structive surgery occurred in this way. I have marveled, in retrospect, that it took so many years for the methods of vascular surgery, so nicely demonstrated by Carrel and others early in this century, to be widely applied in clinical surgery. The principal reason for this was that the patho- logical anatomy of peripheral arterial obstructive disease was so poorly known. Only when curious surgeons, think- ing in actual terms of the disease process in three dimen- sions, began to look into the matter did a flood of new understanding begin. The importance of this kind of curi- osity cannot be overemphasized. Such achievement must be retained at all costs in the atmosphere of the postgrad- uate surgical experience; it represents a point of view to- ward disease which makes surgery an essential at all levels of the undergraduate curriculum as well. It is important to pass on to younger surgeons the quality of intellectual curiosity, but it must first be present in high degree in the staff charged with the development of surgical apprentices.

Although the immediate clinical contribution is abso- lutely vital in a surgical department, it is no longer con-

47

sidered complete by itself. Even in the past, very significant advances in surgery have been made by work done outside of the operating room. Pasteur and Lister with control of infection, Morton and other early anesthesiologists, Landsteiner and blood transfusion, all were towering contributors to surgery although only Lister was a surgeon. The obvious and persistent technical demands of the operation have always tended to place severe limitations on the surgeon's freedom to explore new means of contributing to surgery by activity not directly related to his operation. The grubby realities with which the surgeon appears to deal have often brought disdain upon his head and have led to his being excluded more or less from the refined presence of the physician. The legal wrangles which developed between the College of Master Surgeons and the Faculty of Medicine in Paris in 1748 exemplify this attitude well (and here I have borrowed a quotation discovered by my distinguished predecessor, Dr. E. D. Churchill). I include here a portion of the surgeons' rejoinder to a series of accusations from the Faculty of Medicine in which they sought membership.

Concerning the second indictment, that science is difficult for surgeons and almost impossible for them to acquire, it is said by the Faculty that surgeons do not have the time to study because it is necessary for them to busy themselves to gain manual dexterity in order to operate; further, that it is impossible for them to begin too early to make their fingers nimble. The conclusion is that surgeons should not lose time in their youth with studies. [5]

Fortunately, a full-scale rebuttal to such an indictment is not any longer necessary, and the roots of surgery, which might be thought of as feeding newer possibilities into surgery, are well recognized (Figure 4). These roots are

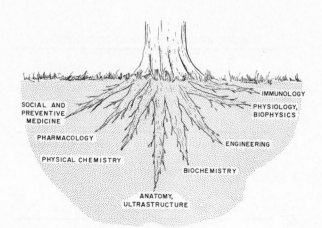

Figure 4. The roots of present-day surgery.

largely common to all the specialties of surgery so that
surgical investigation knows no specialty orientation. The
urologist who is interested in calcification in a stone can
profit by close association with the vascular surgeon who
is curious about calcification in the aorta or the orthopedist
who investigates bone formation. Deep involvement of
many surgical staffs in research of various kinds has occurred, utilizing various scientific disciplines particularly
in the past decade.

A vivid classification of surgical investigation was put
forward by Professor Hedley Atkins of Guy's Hospital at
the time of the one hundred and fiftieth anniversary cele-
bration at the Massachusetts General Hospital (Figure 5).
He recognized that surgical progress could be attributed
to work of three different types and described them as three
tiers of mutually interdependent activity. On Tier I is the
whole realm of clinical observation. This includes all forms
of correlative observations made directly with patients,

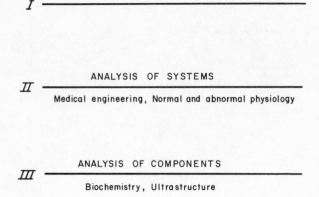

I ──── CLINICAL OBSERVATIONS AND CORRELATIONS ────

II ──── ANALYSIS OF SYSTEMS ────
Medical engineering, Normal and abnormal physiology

III ──── ANALYSIS OF COMPONENTS ────
Biochemistry, Ultrastructure

Figure 5. The three-tiered concept of surgical research, as put forward by Hedley Atkins.

technical innovations in patient care of all kinds, the description of new diseases, and the application of new knowledge to clinical problems. There is no need to emphasize that it is this level of activity which is of supreme importance to all of us in a teaching hospital. Obviously, all the contributions of investigation must be expressed at the clinical level, and many important new leads toward future advances from the laboratory will always develop in the course of patient care.

The properly oriented and motivated clinician-scientist is thus the key to medical progress, but, as I will mention in a moment, there are several varieties of such clinician-scientists who must be nurtured side by side in a teaching hospital.

On the second tier resides activity of a slightly less complex, but perhaps no less difficult, nature. Here organ

50

systems, usually in animal subjects, are analyzed under controlled circumstances. Dogs bark and oxygenators are perfected on Tier II. As a matter of fact, much of the enthusiasm for what might be called more conventional physiologic research has now shifted from departments of physiology to clinical departments where current clinical problems are fresh in our minds and their solution is of immediate utility. Much surgical work remains to be done in the expanding field of bioengineering. Can satisfactory artificial lungs, hearts, livers, or intestines be devised? Can they be miniaturized sufficiently to make them portable either outside or inside the body? Will careful and complete environmental control be a helpful adjunct to certain aspects of medical care? Perhaps we are only at the threshold of major advances in "supportive treatment" at present since we do not yet customarily control the humidity, temperature, bacterial contamination, noise level, and other variables about a patient. With fractional doses of medications and fluids, delivered by monitor-activated and computer-supervised devices, our present intensive care may, in the future, seem almost neglectful. These and other possibilities are already being examined by a collaborative group at the Massachusetts General Hospital, and whether or not much immediate success is achieved, the importance of the team approach to such problems is already established.

On the third tier, the components of living systems are examined. Possessed of a traditional preoccupation with structure, the surgeon is naturally curious about the revelations of the electron microscope when applied to some of his familiar problems. The process of inflammation, the formation of structural proteins, the healing of wounds, the morphological alterations in cells as they begin to mount an immune response, all are examples of such morphological investigations already under way in surgical departments; and, of course, Tier III need not be morpho logical at all.

A modern university department of surgery must therefore depend upon the effort of several different kinds of surgeon, and I want to emphasize that all are absolutely essential to the health of the total enterprise. The expert clinical surgeon may be capable of extending his competence over a fair range of the current clinical front. This is his obligation, but this very fact should give him opportunities, particularly in a teaching hospital atmosphere, which are denied to those with less broad clinical experience. Alternatively, a surgeon may, with appropriate training and background, delve into problems which might be placed on Tiers II or III. In general, his degree of commitment to such activity will tend to narrow his ability to cover a broad clinical region properly, and he will tend to focus on a few areas of special interest. All these surgeons gain mutual strength and stimulation from being in direct contact with one another. The laboratory research surgeon also must work closely with nonsurgical investigators. This is an important aspect of his mission, for he must be the principal means of bringing the flood of new scientific information to use at the clinical level. He is thus the main connection of clinical medicine with the great network of growing scientific knowledge. Since much of his work cannot be expected to be remunerative in fees, he must be paid a salary commensurate with this portion of his work.

What does all this have to do with postgraduate education? Simply that the structure of a department and its staffing make all the difference in the environment in which the young medical graduate matures. People tend to learn by example at all ages, and it has been one of the great assets of the teaching hospital that a variety of living models is constantly before the eyes of each trainee in the persons of a diverse staff. Actual participation in other than clinical research by residents should be optional, and probably only some of those who request this experience should be encouraged. Clinical observations and advances, and the development of a feeling for the depth and variety of the art of clinical surgery, should be the objects of all young surgeons without exception, and the spirit of curiosity and restlessness must be a permanent quality of anyone teaching in medicine today. The constant need for renewal and self-education must be taught in surgery as elsewhere, as we are in constant danger of allowing ourselves to become outmoded. The general nature of this problem was recently emphasized in the *Observer* of London by John Davy in these words:

The basic problem was defined by Lord Bowden, Parliamentary Secretary to the Department of Education and Science, when he said recently that half of what a scientist or engineer learns today will be out of date in ten years. Even a generation ago, a good college training would last a man a lifetime. Now not only technologists but businessmen and many others would benefit from re-equipping every decade — a quite new and formidable educational task which we have barely begun to comprehend. [6]

The Setting of Surgery in a Teaching Hospital. Finally, I come to the newest of the three changes. This has to do with the setting of the teaching hospital and with the influence of great new economic and social factors upon it. Health insurance began to take shape with Bismarck's nation-wide health program in 1883, and extended steadily through Europe, taking the form of government-sponsored plans. Although Lloyd George instituted a National Sickness Insurance scheme in 1913, the complete socialization of Britain's health services came into being in 1948.

We all know of the tremendous growth of health insurance activities in our own country. This response to a growing popular demand will continue; and, aided by the desires of labor unions and employers of all types, including the government, these plans can be expected to join with direct governmental aid to assume the immediate liability for most of the costs of personal medical care. Our patients are no longer wards of society to be placed in ward services (a "ward" is defined in *Webster's International Dictionary* as "a person who, by reason of minority, lunacy or other incapacity, is under the protection of a court . . . or . . . guardian").

This relative affluence represents social progress and a welcome step forward in the fulfillment of the American dream of personal freedom from poverty. The ward services of our teaching hospitals thus tend to be less attractive to the people who previously would have occupied them and to their children. This reluctance is not, for the most part, caused by any conscious feeling by these patients that the standard of medical care on the ward services has been in any way unsatisfactory. It is caused by the workings of our own system of sorting patients into "ward" and "private" on economic grounds. I hasten to say that I do not for a moment dismiss the great effectiveness and importance of an individual physician's assuming continuous charge of a patient's welfare, which has been a feature of medical care more obvious on our private services. This personalized attention is, of course, appreciated by any of us when we are sick and remains a central ingredient in considering the quality of any system of medical care. Pockets of poverty will, of course, persist, and there will continue to be individuals who fit our current definition of ward patients. Teaching hospitals will undoubtedly continue to attract a large percentage of such people in their own communities with the ready availability of specialized help which they represent. Nevertheless, the importance given to medical care by the people of this country is so great that it seems unlikely that the progress of events will leave even those people who might be identified as poor without some sort of financial aid for medical expenses. Willard Rappleye, the former Dean of the Faculty of Medicine at Columbia University, has summarized the situation as follows:

National affluence, public education, prepayment insurance, government participation and other factors are determining that the number of persons receiving medical attention in this country is approaching that of the total population. The amount of services rendered to each individual is also increasing, which is one of the major items in the need for more and better prepared doctors, and more resources such as hospitals, nursing homes, ambulatory care, preventive medicine and rehabilitation. [7]

THE TEACHING OF SURGERY

Let us now focus particularly on the impact of these changes on surgery in a teaching hospital. The hospital is increasingly busier and runs a significantly higher occupation rate, or census, of patients than it did only a decade ago. The operating rooms, constructed for a less surgically oriented institution, are under heavy use, and there is pressure to increase their number and their readiness to provide for complicated surgical operations. Meanwhile, that segment of the hospital traditionally devoted especially to teaching, namely the ward surgical services, has not increased in size. With the tremendous growth in activity of the emergency ward through its attractiveness as a center for the prompt care of acute problems at any time, the ward services continue at a level of activity which is roughly stable, perhaps half of their patient population being derived through the emergency entrance of the hospital. Long waiting lists of indigent patients hoping to be admitted to teaching hospitals for elective operations are disappearing.

On the wards themselves, the patients are older, on the average, than formerly. They represent much more complex problems of care than their predecessors did about seventeen years ago when I began as a surgical intern at the Massachusetts General Hospital. They often have multiple diseases which require the utmost skill and constant vigilance on a twenty-four hour basis, both before and after operation, for any hope of a successful outcome. Their social problems are perplexing and often not really representative of those normally encountered among most patients presently in the private category.

Thus, although the experience of the student and house officer on the ward services remains an abundant one and full of challenge, it has tended to become a somewhat selective one as a consequence of socio-economic changes. There also seems to be little question that for inescapable economic reasons, the number of patients who will come to our teaching services will decline, whether or not large-scale government medical programs are enacted. The setting in which our teaching activities are carried out can accordingly be expected to undergo some adjustments in the fairly near future.

The solution to this problem must involve a realignment of teaching functions without regard to economics. Some teaching hospitals have attempted to expand their teaching function by assuming responsibility for patients in other institutions, such as Veterans Administration hospitals or special state-supported hospitals of other types. This sort of fragmentation would work against the high degree of coherence which the MGH now has; it would tend to disseminate the intellectual growing points of the institution, which will always be closely associated with teaching. It could never be a fully satisfactory solution of the problem of patient supply by itself. I therefore find the notion of some sort of affiliation of this type in order to capture patients for teaching quite unrealistic and unattractive. The patients who must be involved with teaching are here. We have quite enough patients, but we need an adjustment in the mechanism of care of some of them. What are the possibilities? I believe that they can all be brought under three headings:

   I. *Increased emphasis on teaching in our private services;*

  II. *Some means of introducing patients of the private type directly into existing teaching services;*

 III. *The establishment of a new private service especially oriented toward teaching.*

Before considering these possibilities in a little more detail, let me digress briefly to state some of the requirements or desiderata of the medical teaching environment which have emerged from experience, particularly in the past fifty years. Remember, once again, the complexity of the information which is to be conveyed. Remember the structure of the surgical teaching department, which is charged with transmitting both this information and the essential humane precepts which constantly guide its application. Remember the burgeoning of special areas of interest and their common roots in basic clinical principles and in common areas of research.

The core of the whole teaching hospital complex, of all the buildings and all the special facilities, is the teaching ward. One might say that the MGH's soul lies in its teaching wards. These have developed as a splendid arena in which clinical teaching at all levels can be pursued. The environment is not ideal, to be sure, but let us examine its strong points in order to establish the main things which must be preserved at all costs. The ward includes a manageable number of patients, placed under the care of a group of young physicians or surgeons of graded seniority. This group of doctors is a stable one, with the same individuals working together as a team for at least some months at a time. They are closely supervised by senior men of much wider experience who are constantly available for consultation, and who act as guarantors of the quality of the over-all care of the patient. Consultants representing a wide range of special talents are freely available. The ward thus becomes the scene of enlightening discussion and debate. New evidence from the literature and from direct observation is constantly being brought forward. Shared curiosity leads to mutual instruction. Unquestionably, the patient gains. Unbridled curiosity and repetitive questioning and examinations can be a nuisance to a patient, but this can be controlled and is usually overestimated as a hazard.

The provision for some degree of stability of the medical staff, both senior and junior, for certain periods of time is essential to the kind of communication between them which is required for proper teaching. Nevertheless, since apprenticeship of individual trainees should be to the teaching staff of the institution at large rather than to any individual staff member, orderly changes of all personnel are provided.

The continued high quality of all aspects of patient care is kept under constant surveillance, and many checks are provided. The key factor in this entire personal equation is the understanding of each member of the team of his own personal *responsibility*. In the development of a surgeon the growth of his ability to take responsibility is particularly important. Traditionally, the transference of responsibility in surgery has been by an individualized apprenticeship relationship. Although undergraduate medical education has long since departed from this personalized apprenticeship system, such arrangements have tended to linger on at the postgraduate level, especially in surgery and its specialties. The system of postgraduate surgical education prevalent in this country is an American innovation which spread from the Johns Hopkins Hospital to other centers where it has flourished in somewhat modified form. Since the original organization of the residency plan in surgery at the MGH in 1939, one year after the founding of the American Board of Surgery, there has been an increasing emphasis on the gradual assumption of responsibility through the five or six years of postgraduate experience. Using the traditional and perhaps rather superficial measure of who has done the operation as an indicator of where the responsibility on the teaching services of this hospital lies, one finds that it has shifted steadily toward the resident staff (Figure 6). There can be no question that this delegation of responsibility within the group or team has been in no way inconsistent with the highest type of performance in the operating room. Of 97 deaths which occurred in a randomly selected recent year on one of the General Hospital surgical services, only two were considered by the senior visiting surgeons, charged with the immediate supervision of the service, to have been related to the conduct of the operation itself. This figure is a small one and is completely defensible. It emphasizes the fact that the entire management outside the operating room of the kind of complicated problems dealt with on

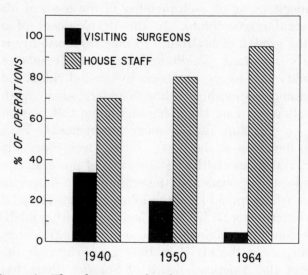

Figure 6. The change in distribution of operative responsibility between house officers and visiting staff on the teaching surgical services of the Massachusetts General Hospital over the past few years.

our services is overwhelmingly the most critical factor in terms of survival. One must point out also that even in the operating room a single individual cannot perform an operation unaided. This fact is becoming more and more striking when in some procedures more than one incision may actually be necessary simultaneously and the patient's life may depend upon the functioning of one or more machines operated by anesthesiologists or heart-lung pump technicians, all of whom reliably assume a certain share of the task. This environment is splendidly suited for the gradual shifting of increasing amounts of responsibility to highly competent and carefully observed younger colleagues. The standard of competence of the entire team is the concern of the senior man; the direct responsibility for the individual details of procedure can, and often must, reside with its individual members.

With these points in mind, let us return to the possible ways previously mentioned by which private patients may become more involved in the teaching process.

First, there could be increased emphasis on teaching within the framework of existing private services. This could certainly be helpful. It is immediately apparent, however, that a group of patients widely disseminated throughout the hospital, under the care of a number of different individual staff members, each understandably and properly preserving his personal relationship with and immediate concern for his individual patient, hardly add up to the teaching environment we seek. Actually, at the present time, teaching on the private services is of the type which depends upon close observation by the residents and upon his participation as an assistant with only modest responsibility. It is generally in a healthy state and makes an enormous contribution to resident education which I do not minimize. No doubt some educational improvements in this area of contact between resident and private patient could be secured, but a high degree of responsibility is not desirable for the resident in situations where the patient has explicitly placed his trust in an individual staff member as his personal physician. Continuity of attention between a resident and individual private patients would be particularly difficult to establish. This method of teaching will continue to be important and has been used to particular advantage in some institutions already, even in surgery. [8] It lends itself best, perhaps, to certain phases of undergraduate teaching where the delegation of responsibility is not so necessary.

The second mechanism mentioned above would admit

certain patients, designated as private, to the present type of teaching service where delegated responsibility is maximal. A number of changes in the service would obviously be necessary before patients, third-party payers, and organized medicine would accept this type of arrangement as the equivalent of what is now considered "private care." The patients would have to be drawn from the increasing number of people who present themselves at the hospital without referral and without any prior personal relationship with a member of our staff. These patients we can call "unmarked private patients." Certain members of the house staff in the more senior years of their prolonged postgraduate experience could be given junior staff appointments. Special regulations could be attached to the privileges granted by such appointments, which would include prior consultation with more senior staff members before certain actions were taken. The outpatient department would have to be suitably rearranged to allow for more continuity of attention by the operating surgeon than is now possible. Private fees would be directed to a hospital fund controlled by the staff and appropriately dispensed for the welfare particularly of the junior staff. A suitable arrangement would have to be made with the accrediting boards so that this supervised experience would be recognized as acceptable. The existing framework of instruction through various meetings, rounds, and close personal attention from the senior staff could be preserved. The difficulties in adapting present services in this way would not be small if the essential features of the fine teaching environment were to be retained.

The final possibility is that some form of intermediate service might be instituted. This new private service would be confined to a particular physical area of beds set aside for the purpose. Certain types of patients, say general surgical and general medical, would be admitted from amongst those coming to the hospital in the "unmarked" category. Senior staff men would be assigned as close supervisors and teachers for given periods of time, but immediate responsibility could be delegated to younger men, perhaps three of four years beyond medical school graduation, who would then be designated junior staff associates. These men would, in turn, be assisted by interns and junior assistant residents. Senior and junior men would function as a group or team with clearly understood responsibilities agreed upon according to the demands of the patient's individual medical problem. Both would normally be present at the time of surgical operation, where the younger man would commonly perform the operation in a manner acceptable to his senior and to the Chief of the Service. Patients would, of course, be freely informed of this. A suitable set of offices in the outpatient department for such "associates' patients" would be required both for initial and follow-up visits. Long-term attention by an individual surgeon would be difficult to arrange under this plan, except in special circumstances, but the quality of the care achievable would be in no way inferior to that available to private patients generally in the community. Fees could be collected by either the senior or the junior men and would accrue to the general benefit of the staff in a suitable way, as salary or in some other form.

Objections to plans of this sort might be expected from four sources: patients, third-party payers, organized medicine, and some of the members of the hospital staff. Patients might possibly object to a reduction in personal attention by a single doctor whom they can trust. Objections on this score need not arise, and actually, as Dr. Russell V. Lee, founder of the Palo Alto Clinic, has said, "The public recognizes and accepts institutional practice more readily than does the medical profession." [9] Organized medicine currently objects to the payment of fees for work done by doctors in training, even though they may be in very advanced clinical training and much better qualified than their contemporaries already in practice who are paid for the same services. It is to be hoped that the threat of competition from institutionalized practice which has caused this stand will wane with time and with persistent efforts to show that in this day of population expansion there will be entirely enough work for all. All segments of the profession must share a substantial concern for the excellence of medical education in the future. Objections from organized third-party payers or group sponsors, such as labor unions, need not be troublesome if the dignity of their members is preserved and their medical needs are discharged with demonstrable and reasonable economy. Finally, the objections of the hospital staff would largely have to do with the strangeness of such a change. If the staff is kept to a size commensurate with the balanced needs of the hospital, and if it is recognized that there is no need or desire whatever to discontinue private practice as it is presently performed, there should be no strong conflicts.

Teaching hospitals are fundamentally healthy because they serve an increasingly essential social function. For us to proceed with our mission in surgery in the most effective way, we must assure the renewal of our ranks with new surgeons seasoned for the changing world in which they will live and work. Our staff must consist of a balanced group of inquisitive and skillful people with differentiated interests, proud of their special vantage point in the world of medicine and of their great capacity to contribute to human welfare. All reasonable provision must be made to allow the many different types of people

— staff, students, researchers, and house officers — to inter-
act with one another as effectively as possible. With these
principles, many lesser problems become easier to examine,
whether they be the question of quarters near the hospital
for the house staff, the unification of the operating rooms in
one area, or the matter of caring for certain economically
independent patients in team fashion.

With these objectives firmly in mind, it is my view that
we can proceed confidently into a rich future.

THE DILEMMA OF MEDICAL
TEACHING IN AN
AFFLUENT SOCIETY

Robert H. Ebert, M.D.

MEDICAL educators have been so preoccupied with the impact of the current scientific revolution in the teaching of medicine that they have had little time to consider the importance of a concurrent social revolution which may be equally important in altering the traditional ways of teaching medicine. There is probably not a medical school in the country which has not made drastic alterations in its curriculum to meet the needs of a changing and enormously expanding body of scientific knowledge. Few have given the equivalent thought to the changing nature of the teaching hospital, and fewer still have thought of the changing pattern of medical care as a factor to be considered in planning the education of medical students, interns, and residents. It is this social revolution which I propose to examine in terms of its impact on the voluntary hospital, the teaching of clinical medicine, and the practice of medicine in the future (as it relates to medical education).

THE DILEMMA OF MEDICAL TEACHING

THE SOCIAL REVOLUTION

John Kenneth Galbraith, in his book entitled *The Affluent Society*, says:

> Nearly all [nations] throughout all history have been very poor. The exception almost insignificant in the whole span of human existence has been the last few generations in the comparatively small corner of the world populated by Europeans. Here and especially in the United States, there has been a great and unprecedented affluence.
>
> The ideas by which the people of this favored part of the world interpret their existence, and in a measure guide their behavior, were not forged in a world of wealth. These ideas were the product of a world in which poverty had always been man's lot and any other state was in degree unimaginable. This poverty was not the elegant torture of the spirit which comes from contemplating another man's more spacious possessions. It was the unedifying mortification of the flesh — from hunger, sickness and cold. [1]

Galbraith's words summarize the nature of the social revolution which has occurred, together with the obsolescence of many of the ideas with which we attempt to interpret the world. Both concepts are important to my theme. It is obvious that the affluence of our modern American society is reflected in the use we make of the hospital today. It is perhaps less apparent that our ideas about the use of the "teaching hospital" are more consonant with the concepts of nineteenth-century poverty than with the reality of our twentieth-century affluent society. There are two points emphasized by Galbraith which are of particular importance in the consideration of the teaching hospital. The first is the support of public service in the affluent society, and the second is the search for security.

In our society those goods and services which can be

sold for a profit represent in aggregate our gross national product, and this is considered to be a measure of how successful we are economically as a nation. Those things which are needed by everyone on a community basis, such as police protection, roads, and schools, are public services and are paid for by taxation. It is not surprising that public services are in general always undersupported. There are too few schools, the police are underpaid, and the building of roads fails to keep pace with the production of automobiles. The hospital is usually considered an instrument of public service, and historically this was precisely what it was, supported either by taxes (the municipal or county hospital) or by voluntary contributions from the community (the voluntary hospital). Today the hospital, while still performing a public service, is financed rather differently, and this is a part of the dilemma which I shall examine a little later.

The second major premise enunciated by Galbraith which is germane to this discussion is the concept of security. How one thinks about security is obviously a relative matter. A factory worker in the nineteenth century who was able to make barely enough to house and clothe his family and who had to worry about starvation if he lost his job would not be much concerned about health insurance or medical care for the aged. His counterpart is very much concerned with these issues because he no longer must be totally concerned with day-to-day existence. It is not the hazard of modern economic life which enforces the search for economic security but rather our general good fortune and relative stability. There are more people predicting the end of the world than the imminent dissolution of General Motors, which suggests that the large modern corporation is a remarkably stable creation. Similarly, the United Auto Workers need not concern itself with the possibility that the union may be broken, but can plan for the economic security and health needs of its members.

The more affluent a society becomes, the more concern there is for individual health, and the greater is the desire to maintain physical health. Sickness and death are no longer accepted as inevitable, and the public comes to look upon medical care as a right and not a privilege. In particular, there are reluctance to accept medical care as a charity and resentment at the idea that one is hospitalized as a ward of the community. Since the major expense of illness is the cost of hospitalization, it is not surprising that the first move to insure greater security for citizens of the community was the development of hospital insurance in the form of Blue Cross. A variety of other insurance plans have been developed, but Blue Cross remains the proto-type of plans which the average employee today expects to receive, whether he pays or his employer pays or both pay in part. The important point of the argument is not so much *who* pays, but rather that insurance has become the accepted way to pay for hospital care by the majority in the community.

The development of hospitalization insurance has had a profound effect upon the teaching hospital, but another change is occurring which may have an even greater im-pact. Once the concept is accepted that medical care is the right of every citizen, it becomes obvious that hos-pitalization insurance does not provide adequate protec-tion. Sickness is an unpredictable expense, and since most care is provided in the doctor's office, the hospital out-patient department, or in the home, hospitalization insur-ance protects only in part against the insecurity of illness. It is natural, therefore, that the concept of prepaid medical care should develop and that it should be fostered by unions. The principle of prepaid care is a simple one. While it may be impossible to anticipate the utilization of medical services by any one individual during the course of a year, such a projection could be made for groups of individuals, and the cost of such usage can be prorated to each member of the group. This means that each member of the group has paid in advance for whatever medical services he requires within certain limitations. The limitations have to do with certain kinds of illness — such as emotional illness — which are still too expensive to be included in such prepaid plans. Perhaps the most successful of these has been the Kaiser-Permanente plan, and the success of this plan and others is likely to bring increasing pressure from unions and consumer groups for this type of protection.

There is one final point that should be made concerning the social revolution before talking about hospitals. By definition, universal poverty no longer exists in the affluent society, but it would be a great mistake to assume that all poverty has disappeared or that it will immediately disappear. There are still pockets of poverty in this country — some of which are rural and many of which are urban. Anyone who has spent time on the wards of the Massachusetts General Hospital, the Boston City Hospital, the Philadelphia General, Bellevue in New York, the Cook County Hospital in Chicago, or the Los Angeles County Hospital can attest in eloquent terms that poverty remains a reality in the United States, and that medical indigency is only part of the problem.

THE HOSPITAL REVOLUTION

The hospital is a social instrument and reflects in rather precise terms the social revolution that we have discussed. On August 10, 1810, James Jackson and John C. Warren

sent a circular letter to several wealthy and influential
citizens of Boston, and in it they argued the need for a
hospital. Several excerpts from this letter are noteworthy:

It is unnecessary to urge the propriety and even obligation
of succoring the poor in sickness. The wealthy inhabitants of
the town of Boston have always evinced that they consider
themselves as "treasurers of God's Country"; and in Christian
countries, in countries where Christianity is practiced, it must
always be considered the first of duties to visit and to heal
the sick. [2]

The letter goes on to urge that it is difficult to properly
care for sick poor at home and to describe the separate
plights of journeyman mechanics, servants, women unable
to provide for their own welfare, and others of the poor.
There is a particularly poignant description of poverty as
follows:

A man may have a lodging; but it is deficient in all those
advantages which are requisite to the sick. It is a garret or a
cellar, without light and *due* ventilation, or open to the storms
of an inclement winter. In this miserable habitation he may
obtain liberty to remain during an illness; but if honest he is
harassed with the idea of his accumulating rent, which must
be paid out of his future labours. In this wretched situation,
the sick man is destitute of all those common conveniences,
without which most of us would consider it impossible to live,
even in health. Wholesome food and sufficient fuel are want-
ing; and his own sufferings are aggravated by the cries of
hungry children. [3]

Quite clearly the MGH and other great voluntary hospitals in this country were founded with the express
purpose of caring for the sick poor. During the first one
hundred years of its history, the MGH was devoted almost
exclusively to this role. A few private rooms were avail-

able, and in 1844 it was decided that patients occupying these private rooms should pay a reasonable compensation for medicine and for medical and surgical attendance. This was set at $3 per week, and all fees collected were given to the hospital to increase the number of free beds for poor patients.

At the turn of the century, there were relatively few private hospitals in this country. Those which existed were of the English nursing-home type designed to provide the creature comforts more than medical facilities. Most people who could afford to pay for medical care were cared for in the home. Most major surgery (for private patients) was done in the home or in small proprietary hospitals.

It is of interest to examine the two major factors which brought about the construction of the Phillips House at the MGH and the provision of hospital care for the well-to-do sick. With the development of asepsis and anesthesia and the founding of special laboratories in the hospital, it gradually became apparent to the wealthy of Boston that the sick poor were receiving better care in the General Hospital than could be provided in the home or in the small private hospital. It was natural that the well-to-do should be interested in the construction of a facility which would provide greater comfort than the General Hospital, but would share in the diagnostic and therapeutic advantages of the hospital. The other factor was the desire to centralize the work of the professional staff of the hospital, so that those physicians who supervised teaching and the care of patients on the wards might be spared the travel required as long as no private facilities existed. It was also noted that a private facility would help to support financially the free beds.

On May 17, 1917, the first private patient was admitted to the Phillips House, and a new era had begun. Because the trustees of the MGH, together with the administrative and professional staff, were the product of a long tradition of service to the community, the next concern of the hospital was provision of care for those of moderate means. It was this that prompted the opening of the Baker Memorial Hospital in February 1930, and the initiation of the so-called "Baker Memorial Plan," which limited the charges made for hospital care and professional fees and which offered care to those with modest incomes who were not eligible for the charity ward but who could not pay the charges of the Phillips House.

The MGH has increased from 458 beds in 1925 to 1,050 beds in 1965. While all parts of the hospital have increased in size, the most rapid increase has been in the size of the private hospital, for this has been necessary to meet the demands of an increasing number of persons with hospital insurance able to pay their way. There is little difference in the expense to the hospital between the patient in the General Hospital and the patient in the Baker Hospital or the Phillips House. Board and room — the hotel part of cost — are relatively minor as compared with the costs which relate to medical care. Therefore the cost of free care or partially free care becomes an increasing financial burden, whereas private care not only pays its own way but helps to a degree support free care. Thus we have two parts of the hospital: one which in a sense sells its service (via insurance carriers in part) and the other which is totally a public service. That part which sells its service can be self-supporting; that part which is a public service is grossly undersupported by the community.

During the past fifty years, and more particularly since the development of hospitalization insurance in the mid-1930's, there has been a remarkable multiplication of community hospitals. By and large these hospitals are for the care of patients who pay their own way, and the amount of free care which they offer is minimal. To compare the financial problems of the community hospital with those of the voluntary hospital is to neglect totally the continuing cost of free care, which drains the resources of the great voluntary hospital. This is a duty of the community unrelated to teaching.

THE TEACHING REVOLUTION

During the seventeenth and eighteenth centuries, medical teaching in this country was accomplished by the apprenticeship system. The likely youth was indentured to a reputable practitioner and by precept learned the art and a very little science of medicine. Beginning in the latter part of the eighteenth century and the early nineteenth century, the medical school was created to supplement the apprenticeship system. In the course of time, however, the teaching hospital assumed the total responsibility for the teaching of clinical medicine, and this custom has continued until the present day.

At the end of the nineteenth century and the beginning of the twentieth century, relatively few hospitals in the country offered continued training after graduation from medical school. The rapid reform of medical education which followed the Flexner Report in 1910 was accompanied by increasing popularity of the internship year. State licensing laws were profoundly influenced by the report, and most states came to require internship training for licensure. Residency training was slower to attain popularity, but the increasing complexity of medical knowledge made more and more specialized training inevitable.

In 1910 there were 24 interns at the MGH and no residents. In 1955 there were 30 interns and 116 residents comprising a total of 146 house officers. Today there are 33 interns and 134 residents, a total of 167.

Prior to World War II, special fellowship training was rare and clinical fellowships were almost nonexistent. During the past twenty years there has been an unparalleled support of research and research training by the United States Public Health Service, and very large sums have been given to support the clinical and research training of young men in the specialties of medicine. There are almost twice as many research and clinical fellows at the MGH today as there are residents (260 individuals).

All of these categories of "students," including medical students, interns, residents, and fellows, depend upon the clinical facilities of the hospital as a resource for their educational experience.

THE DILEMMA OF THE TEACHING HOSPITAL

There is another quotation from the circular letter written by Jackson and Warren in 1810 which is pertinent:

In addition to what has already been stated, there are a number of collateral advantages that would attend the establishment of a hospital in this place. These are the facilities for acquiring knowledge, which it would give to the students in the medical school established in this town. The means of medical education in New England are at present very limited, and totally inadequate to so important a purpose. [4]

A little later the letter states:

A hospital is an institution absolutely essential to a medical school, and one which would afford relief and comfort to thousands of the sick and incurable. On what other objects can the superfluities of the rich be so well bestowed? [5]

Quite clearly the MGH was founded with two ideas in mind: the care of the sick poor, and teaching. It is important to make this point. Traditionally the "teaching patient" has been the "charity patient," and to an important degree this situation still holds. The dilemma which faces the voluntary hospital today is immediately apparent. Its "teaching population" is made up of ward or charity patients, and this group is becoming proportionately a smaller and smaller part of the hospital population. At the same time, the demands made upon the voluntary hospital for teaching are increasing steadily.

THE SOLUTION TO THE DILEMMA

The solution to this dilemma must be apparent to everyone. Either we reduce the amount of teaching which we do (and with the pressure for greater numbers of well-trained physicians this is an unlikely solution), or we use private patients for teaching. This will be difficult to accomplish. Let us examine some of the problems.

Charity patients were used for teaching originally because they were the only patients admitted to teaching hospitals, and it was considered only fitting that in part they should repay the community by being available for teaching. The separation of charity and private care for so long tended to reinforce the idea that only the patients on the wards were suitable for teaching.

If this were the only reason, again, the solution would be simple, but there are other more complex reasons why the use of private patients for teaching is not simple. The patient who would have been in the past a ward patient, and who now has insurance which enables him to pay his way, is likely to think of the role of a "teaching patient" as synonymous with "charity patient." He resents this. He now can pay for the hospital and a doctor and he wants to be treated as an affluent citizen.

At this juncture it might be well to say something about

the clinical teaching of medicine, because if it were simply a matter of the young doctor in training observing the private physician care for his patient, there would be no problem. But this not the teaching method which American medicine has considered particularly effective. Clinical medicine can only be learned well by active participation on the part of the physician in training, and this requires a very real delegation of responsibility. This is a graded responsibility, to be sure, and that given to the medical student is very different than the responsibility given to the intern and resident. Nevertheless, the student participates actively in the care of the patient — always under the closest supervision. The student takes a history and does a complete examination. He does not initiate therapy, by he participates actively in a discussion of the patient's problems, and he may perform various procedures under supervision of the house staff. The important point is that he actively shares in the task of caring for the patient, and he is not a passive observer.

The intern and resident have substantially more responsibility than the student. On the traditional ward service the house officer considers the patients he admits as "his patients," and he must make decisions which involve life and death matters. Everything he does, however, is subject to the closest scrutiny. Each day he (or the student) presents every new patient to a senior clinician who acts as a visiting teacher on the ward, and who has the ultimate responsibility for all the patients in the ward. Two or more hours daily are devoted to this. In addition, the house officer has a variety of expert consultants he can call upon. The two ingredients which make this system work so well are, first, a very real delegation of responsibility, and, second, a critical review of everything which the house officer does.

The system is based on a team approach to patient care which is rather different than the usual manner in which care is provided on the private service. Here the patient's physician carries the primary responsibility, and he may delegate more or less of the responsibility for care to members of the house staff. In the community hospital which has no interns and residents he assumes all the responsibility. In actual fact, in those hospitals which have interns and residents assigned to the private service the house officers must assume an important share of the responsibility at times when the patient's doctor is not in the hospital, but this is often without full knowledge of the patient's problem. The extent of the house officer's authority is often poorly defined since it varies according to the private physician's particular philosophy. The learning experience for the intern or resident is also variable and can range from an excellent stimulating experience to unrewarding drudgery. Ideally the opportunity for the intern and resident to work closely with a skilled physician who is caring for his own patients is an excellent complement to the experience on the ward where he is given more primary experience. But to work well, both the house officer and the private physician must have the time and the desire to exchange views, and to learn from one another. Clearly this cannot be the only kind of experience for the house officer.

The public has a right to ask the question — is the quality of medical care on a teaching ward inferior to the care given in the private hospital? If the answer to this question were yes, then the use of private patients for teaching would be improper, and it is important to add that it would be equally improper to use charity patients for teaching. The fact is that care on teaching wards is as good as the care on private divisions, and in some instances far better.

I will admit immediately that there are certain private physicians who provide superb care for their patients, and that there are some interns and residents who perform below standard, but the reverse is also true and I am talking about a comparison of systems and not individuals. It is far easier to check on the mistakes of an incompetent intern than the mistakes of an incompetent private physician. It is one of the ironies of our system of medicine that a very sick charity patient in the ward is likely to receive better and more constant medical attention than his counterpart on the private side of the hospital.

What, then, stands in the way of freely using private patients in the same manner that ward patients are used? One factor is the reluctance of the patient's private physician to relinquish any of his authority in the care of the patient. He has been taught to assume responsibility and he is reluctant to share it. The patient may feel the same way if he is admitted to the hospital by his personal physician. He feels safer if his own doctor is in charge completely. (It should be noted parenthetically, however, that in a large voluntary hospital such as the MGH many patients present themselves without a physician or are referred to the hospital by outside physicians, and have never been seen before by the private doctors caring for them in the hospital.) A second factor is the doctor's fee. If the physician does not assume full responsibility for the care of the patient in the hospital, he wonders if he is justified in sending a bill.

Neither of these problems is insurmountable. It would be undesirable to have the whole hospital function as a series of ward services. It is in the interest of the teaching service to have portions of the hospital in which the private physician assumes the primary responsibility. Since he is also a teacher, he must have the privilege of practicing in this manner if he is to retain his skills as a clinician, and he must be able to practice in the same environment where he teaches. This part of the hospital service also provides another kind of resource which can be used effectively for certain kinds of teaching. The other problem of fees and how fees are collected is a problem to be solved in collaboration with third-party payers such as Blue Shield.

It should be said at this juncture that a number of universities have built hospitals in which almost all patients are private and all are available for teaching. This usually works well at the medical student level, but problems arise in the delegation of responsibility to house officers. Too often the intern or resident has little more responsibility than he has in the community hospital, and there has been a failure to recreate the teaching environment of the general hospital ward.

Several important principles emerge from this discussion:

1. All patients in a teaching hospital should be available for teaching. There is no point in denying to certain patients the privileges of being used for teaching.

2. There must be a balance between the portions of the hospital in which the teaching team assumes the role of primary care and that in which the personal physician has the primary responsibility. This should not be based on ability to pay, however. Since excellent care can be provided in either area, the quality of care does not become the overriding problem. The idea that only charity patients are to be used for teaching is no longer tenable either morally or economically.

3. All members of the staff must be teachers and involved in teaching. It is anticipated that they will be excellent physicians, but this alone is not enough to justify membership on the staff.

THE FUTURE

I have spoken at length of the enormous changes which have occurred in voluntary hospitals as the result of the social revolution in our society. It would be naïve to think that these changes are at an end, and we can easily identify a number of forces which reflect the increasing demand of an affluent society for better health services, and greater security in the financing of health needs. The pressure of these forces will produce further profound changes in the voluntary hospital and will impel us to alter our traditional views about the use of private patients for teaching. Indeed, it will cause us to re-examine what we teach.

The hospital is changing from a place to hospitalize the sick into a health center, and the forces which I shall mention will accelerate this change. Let me illustrate the point by using the emergency room as an example. The emergency ward at the MGH had its origins in the creation of an ambulance service in 1873. The hospital ambulance would be dispatched for cases of "accident or urgent sudden sickness not contagious, to this Hospital." [6] Obviously the intent was to care for critical emergencies. If we examine the usage of emergency rooms in general hospitals throughout the country during the past thirty years, a striking and constant increase is evident. This is not the result of a parallel increase in the rate of accidents or critical illness, but rather a redefinition of usage made by the public. The emergency room is the place where twenty-four hours a day, care can be obtained no matter what the urgency. The public has made this redefinition because (a) transportation is not a problem; (b) the hospital is always open; (c) it is easier to find a doctor at a hospital than any place else: (d) all the necessary equipment for diagnosis and treatment is available at the hospital; and

(e) many health insurance policies cover visits to the emergency rooms.

Another force which is likely to alter the character of the general hospital is prepaid medical care. I indicated earlier that the concept of prepaid care is a natural one in an affluent society if groups of individuals decide that total health care should be readily available, and the expense should be predictable. It is evident that any prepaid program must have an ambulatory facility, and it is logical that such a facility should be in or near a general hospital so that the complex and expensive facilities of the hospital can be used for the care of ambulatory patients. If such a facility were planned in a teaching hospital without considering how it might be used for teaching, we would further compound the teaching dilemma.

I will mention only one other force which is likely to alter the nature of the voluntary teaching hospital, and that is Medicare. What effect it will have on our teaching wards is unclear. At present almost 50 percent of the patients on the medical wards of the MGH are over 65 years of age, whereas 25 percent of the medical patients in the Phillips House (private) and the Baker Memorial (semiprivate) are over 65. Will many of those over 65 years of age now on the medical wards seek private care, or will they return to the General Hospital and provide additional support financially for the present teaching service? The answer to this question is of enormous importance. The problem represents an additional reason why plans must be made to separate the economics of care from teaching needs.

All of these forces will tend to change the general hospital into a health center responsible to the community for the special needs of some and the total health needs of others. Preventive medicine will become as important as acute curative medicine, and the training of the physician must reflect this changing pattern of health care.

CONCLUSIONS

It is clear that private patients must be used for teaching if medical schools are to survive. It is equally clear that this entails no sacrifice in the quality of care; indeed it insures better care. To be successful, however, it does entail the preservation of the teaching ward environment without a means test. It is totally indefensible to make the ability to pay a criterion for how a patient participates in a teaching program, and planning for the needs of our future physicians will be far simpler once we are rid of this idea.

MEDICAL SCHOOL, TEACHING HOSPITAL, AND SOCIAL RESPONSIBILITY

Medicine's Clarion Call

John H. Knowles, M.D.

IN 1835, De Tocqueville wrote, "In America the passion for physical well-being . . . is general," [1] to which R. M. Titmuss has added more recently, "the larger the investment by any society in 'individualism' . . . the more may 'health consciousness' spread," and "as society becomes more health conscious . . . the more may each individual become dependent . . . in an age of scientific medicine, on other individuals — on resources external to himself. . . . The high esteem of psychology and science in the American culture both emphasizes and expresses this sense of dependency in the search for good health. . . . In relative terms, the individual may come to feel more dependent on psychotherapy, on medical science, on the doctors; less on his own inner resources." [2] There is much evidence of increasing dependence on drugs, doctors, and hospitals as judged by the increasing utilization of all three. Be that as it may, health has become a basic human birthright in America, and like other birthrights, it is being

identified by increasing numbers as a function of government. In the report of the National Advisory Health
Council to the Surgeon General (1961), the statement is
made, "A healthy citizenry is not only a nation's most important 'natural resource,' but also a prime aspiration of
any government whose effectiveness is defined in terms of
its ability to serve the best interests of all the individuals
who compose the society." [3]

Simultaneously society has become progressively more
knowledgeable about its birthright of "good medical care."
Every major newspaper and popular magazine has its own
or a syndicated medical columnist; home medical manuals
and dictionaries abound; hardly a day goes by that the
citizen isn't bombarded by information and advice regarding his health wants and needs; television sends its beam
of psychiatry, neurosurgery, and aspirin into every American parlor and bedroom; and every citizen reads the medical fund-raising material of a hundred maimers and killers.
The contemporary American has the same passionate desire for good health that possessed our ancestors, but now
he has far more insight and an increasing ability to understand medicine, its successes and its failures, as it relates
to his wants and needs.

A sampling from the *New York Times* of Sunday, February 16, 1964 shows the number and range of problems
presented to the public. The headlines read

MENTALLY ILL PUT AT 23% IN NEW YORK
MAINE TO EXPAND ANTI-SMOKING AID
CARE FOR THE AGED — JOHNSON'S PLAN TO PAY MEDICAL COSTS
 THROUGH SOCIAL SECURITY EXPLAINED
WOMEN EXHORTED TO KEEP MAN SAFE — MANY WAYS ARE
 LISTED FOR PREVENTING ACCIDENTS
POLICE CHIEF REVIVES VICTIM OF HEART ATTACK, THEN DIES
SMOKING REPORT TROUBLES NORTH CAROLINA CHURCHMEN

JOHN H. KNOWLES, M.D.

Pregnant Thais See Evil in Many Omens
Narcotic Addicts Find a Cure through Religion
Sister is Certain Ruby was Insane — Suggests "Test of His
   Heart" to Show How He Felt
Electric Larynx Enables the Voiceless to Speak
State Fears Rise in Welfare Roll
Britons Debating Scientist Drain — Exodus a Political
   Issue as Nation Demands Remedy

The basic social issue confronting medicine today is how
to improve the organization, distribution and utilization of
the fruits of medical science and technology, and how to
finance and perhaps even contain the inexorably rising
cost of medical care. Steadily rising hospital costs have
attracted the attention of one and all and have provided a
clarion call to action for our political and union representatives. A recent article in the *New York Times* is typical:

Ribicoff Critical of Hospital Costs
Warns of "Hollow Victory" in Medical Research

Albany, October 3. Senator Abraham A. Ribicoff tonight put
the high cost of hospital care as the No. 1 health problem
confronting the nation.
"If contemporary medical marvels are priced out of the
range of the average American," he said "our brilliant conquest
of so many illnesses will prove to be a hollow victory." [4]

The public is following this clarion call, and the political
trumpet sounds a certain and *not* an uncertain note. This
issue represents common ground where teaching hospital
and medical school interests converge. In order to meet
the problem, provide effective solutions, and determine
the direction of change, teaching hospital and medical
school and their special, mutually beneficial and interdependent roles must be understood and combined rationally. To date, the academic microcosm has appeared to be

uninterested in the socio-economic problems of hospitals and medical care, as judged by the content of curricula and the knowledge of professors of the clinical departments. Too often, professors and deans have looked upon hospital trustees and directors as "just businessmen worrying only about money." In turn, trustees and directors have criticized the medical faculty (and the medical profession) for their lack of social responsibility and their disregard of the socio-economic crises that face the public and the teaching hospitals today. Overhead, some politicians and elements of the state and federal bureaucracy circle the battlefield waiting to pick up the pieces, preying and subsisting on the hopes and fears and lack of knowledge of the voting public, all to the detriment of the medical world. The politician is not entirely to blame. He has received no clarion call from the medical profession except for more federal money for biologic research and less governmental intervention in the financing of health services.

Before discussing in detail the current crisis and suggested solutions, I should like to discuss the threads of administration, authority, and responsibility which bind teaching hospital and medical school together and allow each one to function optimally. Strong administrative and organizational arrangements are necessary if these two institutions are to function effectively in their ultimate role as social instruments. It is well to remember, however, that organization charts do not run institutions, nor do committees conduct research or take care of patients.

MEDICAL SCHOOL AND TEACHING HOSPITAL ADMINISTRATION

Medical administrators occupy exceedingly difficult and highly complex positions in contemporary society. The reasons are simple and revolve around two areas: (1) problems within and peculiar to the medical profession, and

(2) problems caused by lack of public understanding as to the role of medicine and hospitals and those attendant upon our country's own peculiar system of values.

Problems within the Medical Profession. First and foremost as a problem in medical administration is the individual doctor himself. As W. M. Dixon has said,

> The most troublesome thing in the world is the individual man. If anything is in evidence, he is in evidence, and the varieties of this creature are without end. Many are the races and many the temperaments. Who will enumerate them? There are vehement and hot-headed men, selfless and conciliatory men. There are sybarites and ascetics, dreamers and bustling active men of affairs, clever and stupid, worldly and religious, mockers and mystics, pugnacious, loyal, cunning, treacherous, cheerful and melancholy men. There are eagles among them, tigers, doves and serpents. They display, varying as they do in appearance, talents, behaviour, every type of unpredictable reaction to their surroundings. "He was a comedian on the stage," said the wife of a celebrated "funny" man, "but a tragedian in the home." [5]

Doctors, administrators, professors, and employees fit all these adjectives, and those not prepared to enjoy such an array of individuals should maintain their sanity in the various other roles available in medicine and hospitals.

The doctor, however, is unique as an individual and for several distinguishing reasons. Trained to a highly individualistic role, to take immediate action, to give orders which must be followed, and to expect immediate rewards — emotional, financial, or intellectual — he does not always function well as a social animal, where group interest subjects individual interest, no one gives orders which are automatically followed, and rewards are long in coming and must be shared. There is a marked contrast between the interaction of physician and patient versus that of physician and committee or physician and administrator. As Everett Hughes has said, "The queen of the professions, medicine, is the avowed enemy of bureaucracy, at least of bureaucracy in medicine when other than physicians have a hand in it." [6]

Max Weber coined the term "charisma," a theological term meaning "gift of grace," to refer to individuals who exercised authority by virtue of followers who held them in awe and believed them to possess certain special powers. Weber realized that the physician is a charismatic individual and that such individuals are characteristically defiant of administrative regulation and resist the confines of bureaucratic organization. [7] When we are sick, however, the very characteristics of the physician which can make life difficult for the administrators may save the life of the patient. I am sure that Weber would have included a new professional group, the scientists, as possessed of charismatic authority. Again, a certain amount of charisma and a high degree of individualism are very desirable. Professors, doctors, and judges are not expected to march to the mandate of the crowded public forum, although they should keep one ear open to it.

The medical profession is perhaps the classic example of a disorganization that has achieved considerable success. Perhaps the key lies in the intellectual wealth that is recruited, coupled with a certain amount of healthy resistance to change which disappears only when the facts and a logical argument call for change. (Socio-economic facts have *not* produced change from within on the part of the profession, however.) Medical administrators frequently spend time arguing defensively that there *is* a need for administration in medicine, other than the chores of housekeeping, elevator operation, and parking lots. Granted that the authority or the charisma, of the physician and scientist makes the job particularly difficult and indeed defines the need for administration, one may ask, but what else compounds the problem?

The phenomenon of "multiple masters," with resultant dilution of necessary commitment to the over-all institutional welfare, is a factor of major importance. Examples are the practicing physician depending on and answering to his clientele while viewing the hospital as his own host. His own concern has been for the welfare of his patients and rightfully so. He has not, however, had even a secondary concern generally for the hospital as a *social* instrument and today knows almost nothing of the hospital's problems and has therefore defaulted in his position of real power in the community. Physicians *join* the catcalls directed at hospital costs and "inefficient management" and more often than not agree with their patients' complaints. How can they disagree when they have no knowledge? The medical profession generally speaks with authority on the socio-economic problems of medicine; paradoxically, some physicians may be less widely educated on these subjects than the lay public because their education has the limitations of inbreeding and fear of change. Lest the hospital administrator enjoy this tirade, let me say that he has made no attempt to educate his staff and explain the hospital's peculiar problems. Hospital administrators can be just as difficult as any other group entangled in the web of special and vested interests. A promising recent development has been the challenge to responsibility laid down by the American Medical Association's Council on Medical Service, with the advice that the medical staff be considered an integral part of the administrative team. This implies necessary knowledge of administrative problems and the assumption of responsibility — worth-while developments, to say the least. [8]

Another example is the scientific establishment, which has now achieved the status of a profession. The masters of the scientific establishment are the federal government and the National Institutes of Health, and they have generally done a creditable job. The corridors of power have changed, however, in the past twenty years, and the scientists of many a medical school and teaching hospital look now to Washington and not primarily to their own institutions for direction as well as rewards. This represents a massive shift of power from voluntary institutions to the federal bureaucracy. I cannot believe that this is *all* good, what with such problems as inadequate reimbursement for the indirect costs of research, excessive emphasis on biological research, and the current furtive attempts at "effort reporting." On balance, the results have been desirable and the system of decision making excellent. Certainly the postwar expansion of medical research would have been impossible without federal support.

A not so admirable example of the autonomy enjoyed by the scientific establishment is the mass exodus in early 1964 of the Department of Physiology at the University of Birmingham, England to the Worcester Foundation in Worcester, Massachusetts. The *New York Times* of February 16, 1964 states of Professor Bush, Head of the Department, that

At Worcester he will have a guarantee that he will continue to get all the resources he needs to carry on his research. He will also have no administrative problems and no students to teach except when he desires. [9]

Is this the new-found millenium for the scientific profession? I leave it to you to judge its virtues. One further note in the same report states:

JOHN H. KNOWLES, M.D.

A full professor in Britain might earn $10,000 a year. There are great variations in American universities, but some have lured British professors away with salaries not much under $30,000.

All on Professor Bush's team are looking forward to brighter futures. They are impressed by the number of foundations and institutions to which they can turn if they develop research projects of their own. They admire the sheer size of the American Scientific effort.

There is little question that the scientist is achieving a position comparable in status, pay, and charismatic authority to that of the physician in the eyes of the nation, and these two powerful groups tax the ability of the medical administrator to lead or direct. The classic, paradoxical divisions of authority and responsibility that exist in hospitals between practicing staff and director and in medical schools between the "basic scientist" and dean have delighted the sociologist but plagued the administrator.

Personally, I am not pessimistic or even overly concerned with what the head of the Markle Foundation has termed "the low place of the administrator in the spectrum of respect and honor." It may be true that "medical school faculties do not believe direction and leadership are necessary in academic medicine. In fact, they act as if they resent leadership and believe that medical schools should run on an every-man-for-himself basis. They seem to believe that medical schools are free-for-all institutions and not a team operation in any sense of the word." [10] True enough, in some instances, but not all. The statement merely describes the charismatic individual. It invites none but the hardy and capable into the jungle of medical administration.

The dean with his "basic scientists" and the hospital director with his chiefs of service and practicing staff share the mutual problems surrounding charismatic authority and multiple mastership. Heaped upon this is the granting of tenure, which to some means not the freedom to profess one's beliefs openly without fear of reprisal but instead becomes a license for the libertine to act irresponsibly. [11]

To summarize, medical administration is difficult. It is designed not for the faint hearted, the inarticulate, the immature, those seeking power or those who have failed in practice or research. It concerns itself with the activities of highly intelligent, usually highly motivated individuals, possessed of charisma, multiple masters, and tenure. It calls for giant men to provide leadership for such people, to set the scene for their work, and to forge constructive, adaptive change for society at large.

Problems Caused by Lack of Public Understanding. Let us assume that the dean and the hospital director understand the faculty of medicine and the practicing staff, and are successful in coordinating and directing their various energies toward agreed-upon goals with the minimal expenditure of energy and resource. The problem confronting the medical administrator then becomes one of articulating his institution with the wants and needs of society at large. The medical school may be more concerned with defining and, indeed, creating the needs through research and teaching, rather than being directed by social pressures, and the teaching hospital should be more concerned with providing for public wants in terms of direct service. In either event, both institutions are to my mind social instruments whose chief ultimate function is to provide for the health wants and needs of society at large. The means to this end differ considerably, as we shall discuss later.

The major problem that the private medical school and the voluntary teaching hospital face is the public's lack of knowledge and understanding. As a result, crucial moral and financial support may fail the private institution. State and federal medical institutions have similar problems annually when the subdivision of the tax dollar is decided by the politicians. Certainly, there is little or no understanding of why hospital costs are so high, particularly those of teaching hospitals, and are inevitably going to be higher. Similarly, the public knows nothing of the expense of medical education per se. This is medicine's prime failure — that of not educating the public properly about their medical institutions. The future of a democracy and its institutions lies in a citizenry which is adequately enlightened so that it can make choices based on knowledge and understanding and give implied direction to elected public officials. In recent times, the tyranny of short-term, selfish interests has given thoughtful citizens cause for alarm in many spheres of activity, including medicine.

Too often medical faculties have focused so sharply on biological research that the applications of the fruits therefrom have been neglected and left unstudied. Crucial decisions are left instead to the whims of the financially hard-pressed politicians, (lay) representatives of the third-party payers, and an unenlightened but highly vocal segment of the public interested chiefly in cost and not value. Doctors and scientists are perhaps the worst examples of failure when explaining their interests, their values, and their wants and needs. "Think like a wise man, but communicate in the language of the people" is good Aristotelian advice seldom heeded by the medical establishment. Occasionally the problem is not one of inability to speak the language of the people so much as it is the tendency to the smug Olympian view and an understandable but unpardonable reluctance on the part of the university to involve itself in contemporary social issues, except as objects of study. The foregoing is particularly true of the medical school. This comfortable position, occupied by university elite since the time of Plato, is, I believe, going to change in the last half of the twentieth century. It will have to, if medicine is to continue to play the major part in shaping its own future.

Our country's own peculiar cultural attitudes have given administrators a set of public values with which to deal, which must be understood if public support for planning is to be obtained and change is to occur guided by the proper assessments of a community's health wants and needs. Some of these are (1) a traditional deep suspicion of intellectuals, an "anti-egghead" feeling, coupled paradoxically with a respect for the sanctity of the university and its professors; (2) a credit-minded, "satisfaction-guaranteed-or-money-back" attitude; (3) a general acceptance of the concepts of state and federal social welfare programs, and a neglect of local philanthropic giving (for example, local, private funds are given for medical research and capital expansion of hospitals, but very rarely today given unrestrictedly to cover the cost of caring for the indigent sick; county, city, state, and federal welfare is expected to do this through collected tax revenue); (4) a desire generally on the part of the American public to have continuity of medical care, personal care, and technical competence — a culture which, as we have noted, places a high value on health, psychological theories, and science; (5) a tendency for the values of the "rugged individualism" of the past to be supplanted by more concern for social security and a desire for governmental regulation; (6) a deep and abiding suspicion of authority — the idea that "power corrupts" is deeply ingrained in the American mind; (7) the belief that change is good (even though resisted) and that "it's gotta be big to be good";

95

(8) the feeling that achievement is good and that frenetic physical activity per se denotes attempts to achieve, all of which should be carried out with an air of optimism and a "things are great," "keep smiling" appearance; (9) a great need for a feeling of togetherness and belonging, which implies a strong tendency to conformity; (10) a strong time or future orientation; being on time is more important than being polite, just the opposite of South American culture; (11) a belief that depressions are no longer possible because the government, if necessary, would even stockpile automobiles to avert such a disaster, [12] and (12) a desire for good cars, good roads, good defense, good babies in good suburban homes, good health, and an increasing number and variety of services such as education, mass transportation, motels, and hospitals. [13]

As Riesman has said,

The age of abundance has its grandeurs and miseries which are both like and unlike those of any other age, and the searching of aims and discovery of motives appropriate to our new forms of peril and opportunity, along with the discovery of ways to institutionalize our collective aspirations, seems to me the fundamental economic and meta-economic task. [14]

MEDICAL SCHOOL—TEACHING HOSPITAL RELATIONS

The medical school has always occupied a unique and sometimes difficult position amongst the graduate schools of the university. Other faculty members have looked upon medicine as a more vocational pursuit than their own scholarly interests. Another source of friction has been the salaries of medical faculty which have diverged widely and far exceeded those in other graduate schools. Deans of medical schools have become increasingly powerful in the university as their budgets have grown, swollen mainly with federal funds, an imbalance which has been a source of stress to the university's administration. Finally, the medical school has been concerned with the development and maintenance of a very expensive, social service instrument — the teaching hospital. The relationship between school and hospital has been an uncomfortable one. No other department of the university has a similar obligation. The business school does not operate a grocery store, nor the school of education a high school. There is considerable question in my mind as to whether any university should own and operate a hospital. I do not believe that universities should operate businesses, nor do I think that they are in the position to resolve effectively certain crucial conflicts of interest involving university function versus community service. Involve themselves with the social issues, yes, but do not subject the budget of the rest of the university to the possible losses of a teaching hospital, nor the hospital's necessary funds for community service to the needs of the biochemistry or the fine arts department.

Medical schools and teaching hospitals are complex social instruments and as such require strong organization to achieve stated goals and to make adaptive change. The processes of communication and decision making require a visible administrative structure which provides efficient functioning while maintaining a climate of maximal freedom so that intellectual stultification and individual apathy due to rigid bureaucracy do not occur.

Clark and Sheps have conducted studies of teaching hospital–medical school affiliations and written thoughtfully on teaching hospital administration. [15, 16] I find myself in complete agreement with their views concerning the various "Eight Key Issues" that must be resolved successfully in order to have a good affiliation for the purposes of undergraduate medical education: (1) the sharing of the common goals of teaching, research, patient care, and community service; (2) the system of joint appointments of medical faculty and hospital staff, with the power to make such appointments residing in the president and corporation of the university and the board of trustees of the hospital, respectively; (3) the selection of house staff by joint action of university and hospital representatives; (4) the giving of responsibility to the medical student for patient care; (5) the designation of *all* patients in the teaching hospital as (potential) teaching patients; (6) the maintenance of the highest standards of patient care; (7) the support of medical research by *both* institutions; and (8) the need for a clear agreement, "preferably in writing."

Furthermore, I agree heartily, as I have implied above, that "it is most advantageous . . . that the university teaching hospital and the medical school be two separate, distinct, but collaborating entities." [17] Even when the medical school owns the hospital, the administrator should report to a (largely) separate board of trustees and work on a peer basis with the dean of the medical school, who reports to the university president and his trustees. Despite lip service to the contrary, the *immediate* goals of the two institutions are not the same and are occasionally at odds. Furthermore, both institutions are sufficiently complex to require two people working full-time with their respective problems, each understanding and fighting for the particular interest he represents, while recognizing the vitally interdependent and mutually beneficial role of the two institutions.

The goals of the medical school are excellence in teaching and research — the teaching of medical students and the conservation and expansion of knowledge, all for *tomorrow's* health wants and needs. The goals of the teaching hospital are, first and foremost, excellence in the care of the sick and service to the community *today*. In instances where teaching and research (or the university function) have dominated the hospital, the attitude has become set that the patient exists for the teaching program and not that the hospital exists for the patient. Selective admitting policies, shabby patient facilities, and deteriorating physical plant, wards, full of special "research" patients, failure (or refusal) to accept alcoholic patients or expand emergency facilities, a two-class system of care with frequent town-gown battles within the walls of the hospital and disregard for the outpatient department — all lead to a demoralized and spiritless institution. Such a hospital will never send its roots deep into the community for moral or financial support as a consequence of having served the *community's* wants and needs rather than just its own. Only recently have some of our medical school research plans included studies of the patient care and community service functions. This type of "applied" research has a better chance of giving something to the community which will improve the organization and distribution of health services. Coincidentally, we have successful counterparts in schools of engineering, such as Massachusetts Institute of Technology, which have done applied research in conjunction with industry without sacrificing the university's ideal.

The teaching hospital's primary goals of patient care and community service can be at serious odds with the university function by virtue of conflicting demands for money and space. In instances where service and financial considerations have been uppermost, teaching and research have suffered from lack of support and the university program has been of inferior quality, leading in turn to suboptimal quality of patient care. I can offer no magic formula for the proper balance of university and hospital function. I do believe that the attitude of the hospital must be geared to its primary function of caring for the sick, and this attitude must pervade the institution and guide its decisions. I cannot agree with the statement made repeatedly today by medical faculty that "A University Hospital should offer long-term patient care to the extent needed for optimum teaching and research which should be its major goals." [18]

There is one crucial area where I believe both teaching hospital and medical school have failed, and this is the area of planning for the health needs of communities. The greatest blame falls on the medical school, for it could have assumed the role of coordinating agent and provided for rational health planning on a university basis, drawing on its tremendous intellectual wealth for help. Demographers, economists, city planners and architects, public health disciplines, sociologists, and so on are readily available and invaluable to such planning. With the median number of affiliations for medial schools lying between five and seven hospitals, certainly some interest could have been demonstrated by now in assessing the medical wants and needs of communities and in bringing about regional planning for health facilities. Instead, university regional planning has concerned itself only with the needs for "teaching material." Perhaps the new Heart Disease, Cancer and Stroke Bill will help to correct these deficiencies. I shall return to this subject later.

Finally, the medical curriculum and therefore the faculty have not kept pace with the presently emerging, major issues of medical care. Almost no time is devoted to the hospital as a complex social instrument, the socio-economic and political problems surrounding medical care today, or to the social history of medicine. As a result, today's medical school graduate is not well prepared to understand himself, the political and social forces which have defined his present position and which will guide his future, and the steadily expanding number of people and institutions upon which he will be dependent while caring for the sick. [19]

THE FINANCIAL ANATOMY OF A TEACHING HOSPITAL

The primary function of the hospital, regardless of the adjective used to designate its character, is the care of the sick and injured of the community. An additional responsibility of the *teaching* hospital is the conservation and expansion of knowledge through educational endeavor and scientific research. The teaching of medical students; the postgraduate training of interns and residents; the support of schools for nurses, dieticians, medical record librarians, physiotherapists, X-ray and laboratory technicians; the conduct of postgraduate "refresher" courses for practicing physicians and teaching conferences open to all physicians on a regular basis; the publication of clinical experience and research findings and the further sharing of knowledge as visiting lecturer, all round out the activities of the teaching hospital and its staff. In such an environment of constant inquiry, high intellectual activity, repeated questioning of the conventional wisdom, constant scrutiny of established procedure, and the rigorous application of the scientific method, the quality of patient care is likely to be optimal. Our country depends on such teaching hospitals for the setting of standards in the best care of the sick and for the provision of the all-too-scarce supply of well-trained doctors, nurses, dieticians, technicians, and so on. The urban, university-affiliated, teaching hospitals are our islands of excellence in medicine. They must be understood, supported, and protected by the community as well as by the profession so that the long-range interests of our community in matters of health and dis-ease will be served in optimal fashion.

The lot of the teaching hospital is not an easy one. There are only a handful of them among the 176 hospitals in the Commonwealth of Massachusetts, and only some 1000 accredited as such among the 7000 hospitals of this country. Generally they are the same ones which carry the greatest burden of caring for the indigent sick and therefore face the constant crisis of financial disaster. The town-gown battle rages on, and the teaching hospital and its staff bear the brunt of the town's attack. The costs and charges of the teaching hospital are the highest of all hospitals, and the explanation, though constantly sought, is still only poorly understood. The teaching hospital is attracting more and more the complicated and severely ill patient or the patient who requires the care of a specialist, special procedures, and the massive and expensive technical facilities of the large urban hospital. The load it shoulders for the community and its smaller, nonteaching hospitals is becoming increasingly heavy.

In its evolution from a passive receptacle for the sick poor in the nineteenth century to a house of hope for all social and economic classes in the twentieth century, the teaching hospital has seen its costs rise so that a two-week stay in 1925 cost less than did one day in 1964 (Figure 1). Individuals and the increasingly powerful organized purchasers and consumers of medical care (labor unions, Blue Cross groups, state and federal welfare) have scrutinized these inexorably rising costs and in many instances have forged improvement in hospital function. In some instances, chronic harassment, personal (political) gain, and the attainment of short-term, vested interest have been the sole ends. At any rate, the public knows altogether too

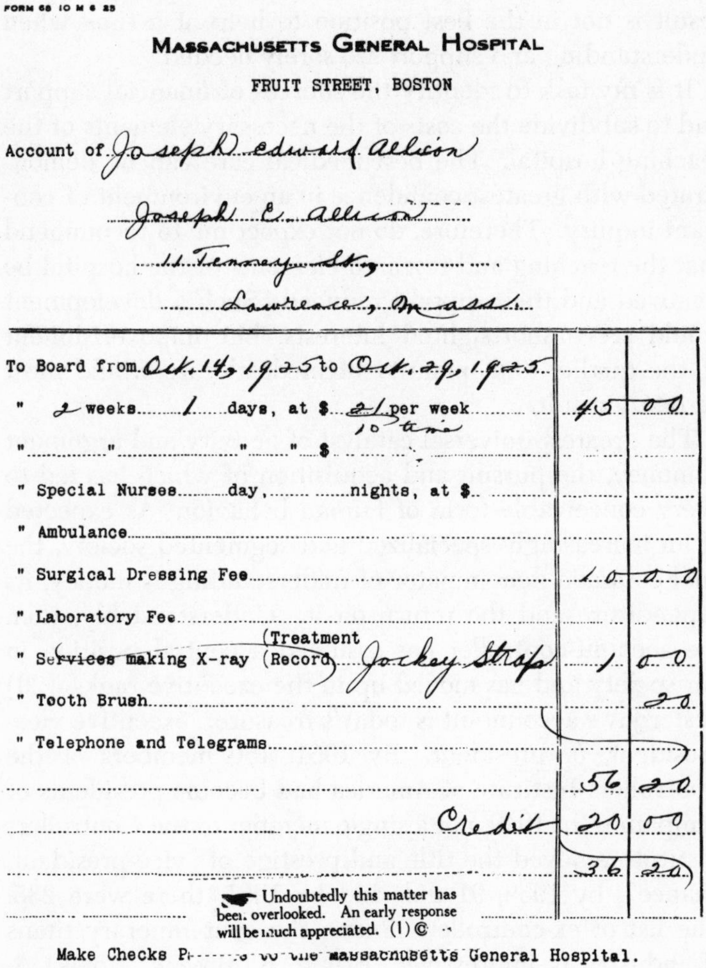

FORM 68 10 M 6 25

MASSACHUSETTS GENERAL HOSPITAL

FRUIT STREET, BOSTON

Account of *Joseph Edward Allison*

Joseph E. Allison

11 Tennery St.

Lawrence, Mass.

To Board from *Oct. 14, 1925* to *Oct. 29, 1925.*		
" *2* weeks...... *1*.....days, at $ *3/* per week *10 time*	45	00
" .... " .... " .. " .. $		
" Special Nurses.........day, ...nights, at $...		
" Ambulance.........		
" Surgical Dressing Fee.........	10	00
" Laboratory Fee.........		
" Services making X-ray (Record) (Treatment *Jockey Strap*	1	00
" Tooth Brush.........		20
" Telephone and Telegrams.........		
	56	20
Credit	20	00
	36	20

Undoubtedly this matter has been overlooked. An early response will be much appreciated. (1) ©

Make Checks P~~ayable to the Massachusetts~~ General Hospital.

Figure 1. Cost for two-week hospitalization in 1925.

little of the operation and function of its hospitals and as a result is not in the best position to help at a time when understanding and support are sorely needed.

It is my task to identify the sources of financial support and to subdivide the costs of the necessary elements of the teaching hospital. The best medical care can be demonstrated with greatest confidence in an environment of constant inquiry. Therefore, do not expect me to recommend that the teaching and research elements of the hospital be removed and their support reduced. Such a development would serve shortsighted interests, but impoverishment of the quality and quantity of medical care would most certainly result.

The greatest universal catalyst of activity and argument is money, the pursuit and acquisition of which has led to every conceivable form of human behavior. As expected of an increasingly specialized and segmented society, the final common denominator of understanding is money, its expenditure and the return on it. Understandably, then the account-controller has assumed a central position in our society and has moved up in the executive ranks. [20] Yesterday's accountant is today's treasurer, executive vice-president, or president. By 1961, 150 members of the Controllers Institute of America had become presidents of companies. In 1949, not a single member of the Controllers Institute enjoyed the title and prestige of "vice-president, finance"; by 1959, 91 did, and by 1961, there were 235. The list of ex-controllers among the contemporary titans of industry is impressive: Ernest R. Breech, Robert S. McNamara, and Gerald Phillippe, to name but a few. [21]

To turn to our own business, how often do we hear, "What will the auditors say?" or "I don't know what the GAO will think of this!" For indeed, precise and detailed knowledge of the expenditure of the dollar will reflect accurately the functional life of the institution as well as the place it occupies in the community. It can also tell within limits how well it is doing its job. I should like to dissect the financial anatomy of one hospital and trace the subdivided use of its dollars, for herein lie some crucial problems and some broad issues which must be recognized and resolved.

THE DEVELOPMENT OF INDIRECT PAYMENT FOR MEDICAL CARE

Arnold Toynbee has said that the twentieth century will be remembered as the first age in history in which society has thought it desirable to make the benefits of civilization available to the whole human race. In the area of health and social welfare, this has been manifested by the development of employee fringe benefits, brought about by the expansion of unions and the use of collective bargaining; the expansion of organized philanthropy, such as United Fund (Community Chest), Federated Jewish Philanthropy, and such organizations as the American Heart Association and the American Cancer Society; the passage of Workmen's Compensation Laws in 1910, the Social Security Act of 1935, the Kerr-Mills amendment to the Act, and the Medicare amendments of 1965; and the development of Blue Cross and Blue Shield in the 1930's, as well as the expansion of commercial insurance companies.

Practically speaking, nearly all these developments occurred or were accelerated during the 1930's, following the Great Depression which "began officially" October 23, 1929 with the stock market crash. With the election of Roosevelt and his accession to the presidency in March 1933, the federal government received the mandate to relieve the situation and thus began the present era of deficit spending and federally supported social welfare programs. [22] The great debate of those wishing to preserve the values of individual initiative and self-reliance at the expense of social welfare programs, and vice versa, began then.

Prior to the 1930's, voluntary hospital bills and doctors' fees were paid directly by most individuals, while private philanthropy through its "unorganized" giving to hospitals supported those who could not pay the bills. City, county, state, and federal hospitals took care of the rest, plus certain chronic illnesses (such as tuberculosis and mental disease). Doctors gave their services freely to the indigent sick.

By 1940, there were established several sources of income to the *voluntary** hospital: the direct paying patient; reimbursement from state welfare departments either under provisions of the Social Security Act of 1935 or under noncategorical state, city, and town relief acts; reimbursement from Blue Cross and commercial insurance companies; endowment funds, annual gifts, and United (Community) Fund or Federated Jewish Philanthropy allocations. In addition, the teaching hospital has one other potential source: the university.

GENERAL FINANCIAL STATUS, 1940 TO 1964

Before we analyze each one of these sources of income as they exist today, the whole picture should be viewed in broad perspective using one voluntary, teaching hospital as an example (see Tables I and II). As we view these figures, bear in mind that the Massachusetts General Hospital today is a 1,050-bed teaching hospital, which in 1964 had a total of 338,244 patient days. Per diem costs can be multipled by this figure to give annual costs for the

---

* The word "voluntary" as applied to institutions dates from 1745, and is described in the Oxford Universal Dictionary as "maintained or supported largely by free will offerings or contributions, and free from State interference or control."

TABLE I. Massachusetts General Hospital Operating Results, 1940–1964 (dollars).

Year	(1) Operating income (net)	(2) Operating deficit	(3) Deficit total hospital	(4) Earned depreciation	(5) Difference between Col. (2) and Col. (3) (roughly equivalent to endowment and other income plus community fund)	(6) Free work, Blue Cross and state welfare agency loss plus provision for bad debts
1940	2,084,000	891,000	171,000	—	720,000	434,000
1941	1,923,000	835,000	43,000	—	792,000	525,000
1942	2,081,000	897,000	93,000	—	804,000	531,000
1943	2,252,000	810,000	31,000	—	779,000	484,000
1944	2,488,000	918,000	126,000	—	792,000	352,000
1945	2,726,000	1,156,000	307,000	—	849,000	360,000
1946	3,162,000	1,174,000	429,000	—	745,000	498,000
1947	3,880,000	1,099,000	244,000	—	855,000	713,000
1948	4,791,000	923,000	46,000	—	877,000	1,052,000
1949	5,384,000	1,109,000	297,000	—	812,000	1,386,000
1950	5,884,000	879,000	80,000	—	799,000	1,137,000
1951	6,603,000	986,000	172,000	—	814,000	1,193,000
1952	6,942,000	863,000	99,000	—	764,000	1,246,000
1953	7,575,000	974,000	(29,000)ᵃ	—	1,003,000	1,347,000
1954	7,934,000	1,479,000	14,000	—	1,465,000	1,473,000
1955	8,658,000	1,318,000	19,000	—	1,299,000	1,896,000
1956	9,723,000	1,501,000	87,000	142,000	1,414,000	1,917,000
1957	10,823,000	1,454,000	44,000	337,000	1,410,000	2,307,000
1958	12,525,000	1,642,000	183,000	482,000	1,459,000	2,473,000
1959	13,840,000	1,517,000	106,000	698,000	1,411,000	2,473,000
1960	15,270,000	1,877,000	477,000	668,000	1,400,000	2,811,000
1961	16,740,000	1,228,000	(281,000)ᵃ	796,000	1,509,000	3,058,000
1962	19,011,000	1,443,000	48,000	930,000	1,395,000	3,416,000
1963	21,269,000	1,434,000	24,000	1,091,000	1,410,000	3,395,000
1964	23,163,000	1,691,000	193,652	1,218,000	1,497,000	4,328,000

ᵃ Figures in parentheses indicate excess of income over expense.

JOHN H. KNOWLES, M.D.

TABLE II. Massachusetts General Hospital, comparison of total deductions from income with United Community Services allotments, 1951–1964 (dollars).

Year	Total deductions from income[a]	United Community Services allotment	Percentage of U.C.S. allotment to total deductions
1951	1,193,000	272,000	22.80
1952	1,246,000	249,550	20.03
1953	1,347,000	255,390	18.96
1954	1,473,000	200,000	13.51
1955	1,896,000	178,617	9.37
1956	1,917,000	190,000	9.91
1957	2,307,000	180,000	7.80
1958	2,473,000	224,620	9.08
1959	2,473,000	226,330	9.15
1960	2,811,000	194,478	6.92
1961	3,058,000	222,481	7.28
1962	3,416,000	160,071	4.69
1963	3,395,000	192,188	5.66
1964	4,328,000	196,400	4.54

a Figures represent the sum of free work, Blue Cross and state welfare agency loss, and provision for bad debts.

year 1964. Costs discussed in this paper refer to inpatients. Outpatient costs have been excluded. Table I shows the operating results of the Massachusetts General Hospital for the twenty-five-year period from 1940 through 1964. There are several important observations to be made.

Expansion of Free Work. In 1940, our unreimbursed expense for patient care (free work, Blue Cross and state welfare agency loss, and bad debts) was $434,000, while endowment income plus Community Fund was $720,000, which therefore more than adequately covered the "free work" of the hospital. In 1964, endowment income had doubled to $1.5 million and "free work" (unreimbursed

108

care) had increased nearly tenfold to $4.3 million, as com-
pared with 1940, and it was necessary to collect over $2.8
million extra (of involuntary money) from the private
paying patients, our only earning asset and remaining
source of added funds. The failure of voluntary community giving and the inadequacy of reimbursement for welfare patients forced us to overcharge paying patients and
their insurance companies to make up the difference.

Operating Deficits. From 1940 through 1964 the hospital
had operating deficits every year save two totaling over
three million dollars. This money had to be obtained by
using unrestricted capital gifts to the hospital or, more
commonly, by reducing the expenditure for depreciation
in the ensuing year. Using these monies, plus virtually all
endowment income (for "free care"), left nothing for
capital expenditures (or "venture" capital), which therefore had to be raised through special annual drives. I note
with interest that the formerly voluntary hospitals of
England have been allowed to retain their endowment
and are required to use the income for capital expenditures
in the main. They are *not* allowed to use it to cover
operating deficits.

United Fund Allocation. By agreement with the United
Fund, the hospital conducts its annual fund-raising drive
only during the month of December, to lessen the competition for money. In many ways this is a direct financial
contribution to the Fund, for the MGH could raise more
money if allowed to solicit in the Greater Boston area the
entire year. In return for this demonstrated "good citizen-
ship," how have we fared with the United Community
Services allocation? (UCS is the division of the United
Fund in Massachusetts concerned with health and hospital

problems.) A glance at Table II shows that in 1951, we received $272,000 from this source, which was equivalent to 22.80 percent of our total deductions (unreimbursed care). In 1964 we were given $196,400, or 4.54 percent of total deductions, representing a steadily diminishing allocation from the UCS over the years. This is mute and incontrovertible evidence of the failure of coordinated voluntary, community giving to keep up with the needs of teaching hospitals, at least in Massachusetts.

Depreciation. In 1956, the MGH began earning and funding depreciation, and we remain one of the few hospitals in the Boston area which is able to earn its stated depreciation. In 1964, we earned $1,218,000 and spent it entirely on maintenance, alteration, and renovation of our plant, and the repair and replacement of equipment. What happens to hospitals which don't fund depreciation and spend it, or are unable to earn it? The plant and equipment crumble, the operation becomes extremely costly, and the best ultimate decision is to abandon the ship and hope for good salvage income. Listen to these comments by a New York City hospital director:

When I first came here five years ago, practically no maintenance or modernization work had been done for years. Any money the hospital raised had gone to meeting deficits caused by low Blue Cross rates and low city fees for ward patients. . . . We are making a strenuous effort to mend and modernize. . . . A new thoroughly modern kitchen has been installed . . . at a saving, incidentally of $175,000 a year. [23]

It has been estimated that it would cost more than $185 million to bring New York's voluntary hospitals up to the proper standards for safety. [24] A recent study of the Boston City Hospital states that it would cost more than $45 million to bring its plant up to snuff over a twelve-year period beginning in 1963, [25] and in 1963 a special appropriation of $2 million was needed to build up the Radiology Department so it could be accredited.

Hotel versus Professional Cost. The cost per day at the MGH has risen from $10.25 in 1940 to $50.10 in 1964. This increase in cost is typical of the large, urban teaching hospitals of this country. Recently our expenses have increased at an annual rate of 6 to 7 percent. It is clear to all that, as medical science and technology has expanded, the subdivision of medical labor has increased. The rapidly rising cost of hospital care is due to the "professional care" element (those things and people one needs in a hospital but not in a hotel) and not to the hotel function. Three-quarters of patient income goes into the salaries of our employees, and most hospital workers remain grossly underpaid in this country. At the MGH in 1964, 11.6 percent of the dollar was spent on "hotel function" and 88.4 percent on the professional or medical function, as contrasted with 28 percent and 72 percent, respectively, in 1952 (Figure 2). The two pie charts in Figure 2 bear careful scrutiny by *all* interested in medical care; they demonstrate first and foremost the expansion of medical technology and specialization. *The most important consideration is the fact that the medical profession controls potentially the expenditure of 88.4¢ on the dollar.* The administrator controls the 11.6¢ and perhaps another 30.7¢ representing the expenditure for the nursing service. Here lies the traditional dilemma of the hospital director — he is responsible for the total cost of hospitalization, but has clear-cut authority over only 10 to 40 percent of the expenditures. The medical profession generally has exercised authority in the 60 to 90 percent area *but* has not carried the necessary responsibility.

111

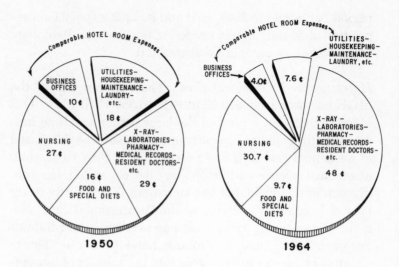

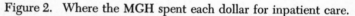

Figure 2. Where the MGH spent each dollar for inpatient care.

THE SOURCE OF INCOME

With this information in the background, let us review the status of each one of our sources of income and describe the dilemma we face. In 1962, the nation spent $31.7 billion for health care, or $170 per person. Three-quarters, or $23.8 billion, was spent by private individuals or agencies, and one-quarter, or $8.0 billion, was spent by the government. The largest single item by far was the expenditure for hospital care — $10.5 billion, of which $9.1 billion was for care in nonfederal facilities. [26]

In Table III we have shown our own experience for the years 1962 and 1964. The table is self-explanatory.

Some observations are necessary here about each one of the sources today, for verily, he who pays the fiddler *will* call the tune.

The Private, Direct Paying Patient. As we have noted,

TABLE III. Source of Massachusetts General Hospital Inpatient Income, 1962 and 1964

Source	1962	Percent	1964	Percent
Consumer[a]	$ 5,339,000	37.9	$ 4,473,000	26.3
Blue Cross	4,318,000	30.7	6,092,000	35.8
Commercial insurance	1,783,000	12.7	2,394,000	14.1
Welfare	1,248,000	8.8	2,553,000	15.0
Endowment income	1,395,000	9.9	1,496,000	8.8
Total	$14,083,000		$17,008,000	

[a] Consumer income comes from direct paying patients and those who hold co-insurance contracts where they are liable for part of the bill.

prior to the 1930's most individuals paid their own hospital bills directly. This method of payment had distinct advantages from the standpoint of public education and understanding — questions were asked and answered concerning the bill. The number of individuals today in this country who have no form of insurance and who pay their own bills directly is *small* and steadily diminishing. The figure is 15 to 20 percent of the patients at the MGH today. Furthermore, this group is apt to consist of the very wealthy, who are self-insurers, and who therefore don't ordinarily haggle about their bills. The opportunity to explain the hospital bill and educate the public is therefore lost. The following statements are common:

The typical hospital patient interviewed did not seem to care about hospital charges since his first three weeks in a semi-private accommodation under Blue Cross cost him nothing.

One man, an elderly bank clerk, said he had had two wives who died in hospitals and that he had been in five hospitals because of a stomach ailment.

"I never looked at my bills," he said, "because I didn't have to pay them. They were covered by Blue Cross. Sure, I got copies of the bills, but I couldn't care less what the costs were." [27]

I believe that this attitude is typical, and the number of comprehensive contract holders is expanding steadily. In Massachusetts it has increased from 18 percent in 1959 to 32 percent of all Blue Cross insurance policies in October 1964. The beneficial influence of an enlightened community of people who have questioned hospitals, learned about them, and perhaps effected change in them through their own experiences has steadily diminished. The first line is now the third-party payer, private or governmental, and he bears the initial brunt of the attack when the rates and premiums have to be raised. He is the hospital's buffer agent, just as the teaching hospital has been the medical school's buffer against the social problems of medicine. I am *not* convinced that these representatives have told the story well, nor are they in the best position to do so. Too often they have merely said "We can't do anthing about it — it's the rise in hospital costs!" and have not seized the opportunity for better education of the public regarding *what* caused the rise! Over the past three years, we have raised the rates at the MGH three times. I have yet to hear a single complaint! — an unheard-of situation just ten years ago, to say nothing of thirty years ago. No complaints, no questions, and an opportunity lost to educate the public. All would agree, however, that the growth of health insurance plans has been totally desirable. A negative element in the aftermath of their expansion has been a decentralization of the community educational function (as well as potential power and authority) from the hospital to outside agents.

Payment by Health Insurance. The 1930's saw the initiation of the Blue Cross plans and the expansion of commercial insurance companies into the field of health. By 1940 some 9 percent of the population had some form of health insurance; by 1962 the percentage had increased to 76 percent of the country's population, or 141 million people. [28] Approximately three-quarters of Americans with health insurance were enrolled through employee benefit plans. Consumers were now organized, and their collective voice has been raised increasingly as collective bargaining for health insurance benefits has introduced powerful consumer groups, mainly union, into the medical care field. Cost of care and its availability, distribution, and quality have been scrutinized increasingly by the organized consumers' elected agent, and the employer, too, has stepped in to see what his fringe benefit expense is buying.

Major medical expense plans have continued to grow rapidly, and nearly 40 million Americans now have this form of insurance. The repeated demonstration that individuals and groups will usually choose the best, most complete and comprehensive coverage, and not the lowest *cost* alternative, when faced with selection of a program, is of extreme importance. This fact, coupled with our own experience that utilization of health facilities is related not primarily to cost but to service, has important implications for medical schools and teaching hospitals.

The Blue Cross plans, of which there are 77 currently in operation in the United States, have usually been well established by state legislative acts because of their voluntary, nonprofit nature. Legislation has usually provided exemption from the insurance laws of the state, description and appointment of governing board, careful inspection of operation and approval of rates by the appropriate state agency, and tax-exempt status. Thus the Blue Cross is very closely scrutinized by the state and subject to various political forces and finds itself squarely in the public eye when approval for rate increases is requested of the state. Having been initiated by a hospital in 1929 and having been guided by and closely allied to the American Hospital Association, the Blue Cross has found itself in the difficult position of trying to determine whose agent it will be. Does it represent the hospitals, functioning purely as a prepayment plan for financing hospital costs, *or* should it represent the subscriber and be his financial agent in controlling hospital costs by scrutiny of hospital operation, insuring complete utilization of services, effecting regional planning, and guaranteeing a minimum quality of care? The Somerses have stated the problem:

> The ambivalence of its current position — midway between a hospital-controlled institution and a public service organization, expected to be equally responsive to hospitals, subscribers, and the public — is perhaps the most difficult problem confronting Blue Cross today and intimately related to its ability to surmount its current enrollment and financial crises. [29]

With every rate increase, the public cries "Help!" and the politicians howl about inefficient, dishonest management, too high salaries for administrators, laxity on the part of Blue Cross and hospitals in containing costs, and so on. This phenomenon, plus the very real problem of resolving its identity as to whose agent it should be, has provided Blue Cross plans with repeated crises. In addition, the future of the whole program has been jeopardized by repeated decisions by the state in times of crisis and/or rate increases which have resulted in more state control.

Finally, the Blue Cross has had an intensely competitive relationship with the commercial insurance companies, [30] which at times has distracted them from their mutual goals and led some to believe that government intervention and sponsorship of health insurance is the ultimate answer. The failure of voluntary insurance plans to solve the problem of poor risk groups, specifically the aged and the medically indigent, has led many to believe that the Social Security mechanism of forced prepayment is inevitably the only rational answer.

As of 1964, commercial insurance usually pays the hospital's charges, whereas Blue Cross contracts, at least in Massachusetts, pay specific costs and not charges. Roughly 40 percent of our patients have Blue Cross insurance while 30 percent are insured by commercial companies. There is considerable overlap here because of double indemnity, however, a condition which is permitted only in health insurance and which allows some people to make money when hospitalized. Our current problem with the Blue Cross in Massachusetts will be discussed below.

Welfare Reimbursement. For the fiscal year ended June 1963, the acute hospitals of Massachusetts received a total of $14,953,620 from public welfare funds, of which nearly $10 million represented reimbursement under Medical Assistance for the Aged and Old Age Assistance (see Table IV). The costs were subdivided among federal, state, city, and town governments. For example, under MAA (Kerr-Mills Act), the federal government paid half of the total, the state two-thirds and the city or town one-third of the remaining cost. In 1962, the MGH received roughly $1.25 million of the total $15 million given to acute hospitals in Massachusetts for the care of the medically indigent population.

The greatest problem with welfare reimbursement from the hospitals' standpoint is the method of its determination, which has *always* resulted in payments *less* than the cost of caring for the patient. The greatest problem from the standpoint of the aged is the necessity for a means test, which may delay medical care. Furthermore, the means test can cost the state as much as $200 to conduct. The

117

TABLE IV. Public Welfare Department expenditures for acute hospitals in Massachusetts, fiscal year 1962–63.

Public welfare categories	Patient days	Cost of total acute hospitalization	Federal government	Share of cost paid by —	
				State	Cities and towns
Medical Assistance for Aged	212,526	$ 4,908,211	$2,454,105 (50%)	$1,636,071 (⅔)	$ 818,035
Old Age Assistance	211,501	5,076,893	924,048 ($54 per case times 17,122 cases)	2,768,564 (⅔)	1,384,281
Disability Assistance	81,096	1,984,464	260,400 ($46.50 per case times 5,600 cases)	1,293,048 (75%)	431,016
Aid to Dependent Children	67,072	1,677,668	215,004 ($20.50 per case times 10,488 cases)	487,554 (⅓)	975,110
General Relief	52,502	1,306,384	—	261,277	1,045,107
Total	624,697	$14,953,620	$3,853,557	$6,446,514	$4,653,549

greatest problem facing the Welfare Department is first and foremost a confusion of its true role, which is to provide help to those in need rather than simply to conserve the budget for those in political power.

The state's Division of Hospital Costs and Finances and the Commissioner of Administration have for years arbitrarily set ceilings of reimbursement, which are always below the hospital's cost of caring for welfare patients. Hospitals in Massachusetts have never received full reimbursement of costs for a variety of reasons, including the limited tax funds subject to other competing priorities, poor understanding of or refusal to understand the necessarily larger costs of teaching hospitals, and, finally, a feeling by welfare agents that their role is served best by being a withholding penurious watchdog and their belief that hospital costs can be kept down if the reimbursement rate is kept down. Furthermore, the administrative practices in setting such rates of reimbursement have been arbitrary, with an inadequate appeal mechanism; they were declared illegal by the Supreme Court in a suit brought by the Massachusetts General Hospital against the state in 1964. The present formula (1966) used by the state for determining reimbursement for welfare patients is guaranteed not to give the hospitals their costs — *ever*.

As hospital costs have risen, so have the costs of caring for the medically indigent, and the losses for caring for welfare patients as well as those losses due to free care have reached staggering proportions. As stated before, endowment funds and those given to hospitals by the United Fund have been far outstripped by such expenses, and the only solution has been to overcharge paying patients and their insurance companies. Some thought this a satisfactory solution until the state, which has comprehensive Blue Cross insurance for its employees, ruled recently that the Blue Cross contract for comprehensive care would allow only costs and *no* added reimbursement to help share the cost to the hospital of "net" free care (that is, that amount of free care not covered by, or in excess of, endowment income and United Fund allotment). This problem, plus that of inadequate reimbursement for welfare patients, has precipitated one crisis after another in our relationship with the Blue Cross, state Welfare Department, the politicians, and the public at large. [31]

Hospitals, particularly in the Eastern part of the United States, have suffered at the hands of evanescent and irresponsible politicians functioning on a short-term basis. Thus, the Boston City Hospital has been reduced from 1800 beds to an active hospital of roughly 1000 beds today. Its physical plant is nearly obsolete and even minimal repairs have been neglected. As noted, a study in 1963 estimated the need for $45 million to bring the hospital up to date. The politicians have squeezed the institution dry — a major teaching hospital of *three* great universities. Has any righteous indignation, or even concern for the proper plant and facilities, been expressed by the universities, their deans and professors? Has the public demanded a first-class hospital and brought effective pressure to bear? The answer is *NO* in both instances. Our political representatives have received no clear mandate from the experts or their constituents. *We* are to blame as much as they.

Consider what has happened to the Jackson Memorial Hospital in Miami, Florida. The *Miami Herald* of Friday, April 17, 1964 headlines the following on page 10-C:

Cost Climb Makes Taxpayer Arbiter of JMH's Future

Jackson: Top Medical Center or Long Slide Downhill?

JMH: Hospital in Crisis

SOCIAL RESPONSIBILITY

Dean Hayden C. Nicholson, in a statesmanlike article for the *Miami Herald*, of the same date said

> The deterioration at Jackson Hospital undoubtedly is due in large measure to inadequate financial support. I am told that the hospital has operated on essentially a constant budget the last two or three years and apparently is expected to do so again next year.
>
> Unfortunately, hospital costs country wide have been rising at a rate of 7 to 10 percent a year for the last decade. Asking a hospital with a constant patient load to continue to operate on a constant budget each year during such a period of rising hospital costs amounts to reducing its budget each year by the amount of the increased costs. Progressive deterioration is inevitable and inexorable.

"Progressive deterioration is inevitable and inexorable" indeed when short-term interests prevail, and the tyranny of multiple priorities on the tax dollar usually finds the hospital on the shortest end of the stick because it lacks sustained vocal support.

In the *Miami Herald* of Sunday, June 7, 1964, County Manager Irving McNayr admitted that the "budget which gives Dr. Gates [Executive Director of the JMH] less than one-tenth what he asked for in increased funds, was prepared under instructions from the Metro Commission to hold the line on taxes." Mr. McNayr was quoted as follows:

> "The real crux of what we are talking about is money," McNayr said. "Are the people willing to pay the money for increased services?
>
> "I'm not opposed to better services. I'd like very much to have the highest level of service that the people are willing to pay for — and that's true also in terms of the sheriff's department, fire protection, streets and all the other county services.
>
> "In the three years I have been here we've had not more

121

than six or eight spokesmen urge more funds for any department. In regard to Jackson, *there has been no citizen demand, no medical school demand . . .* we would welcome it so far as Jackson is concerned." [*Italics supplied.*]

Finally, note carefully this paradoxical situation in the midst of crisis. In the same article, Metro Budget Director Dennis I. Carter

insists Jackson has not been ignored, pointing out that Jackson will get $448,0000 more in the budget than this year.

"That's more than the total increase for the entire county budget," he said. He added that Jackson's proposed budget is $2.3 million more than four years ago, although the hospital is handling fewer patients today than in prior years.

But he admits the increase in funds provided in the proposed budget will come from private patients, not the taxpayers. The hospital is counting on an increase in room rates to help it out of its financial problems.

Taxpayers will be called on to come up with $189,000 less for Jackson during the year. The taxpayer's share of the JMH operation this year is $7,738,319. Next year, it's $7,548,731. [*Italics supplied.*]

This situation is so similar in many respects to our own that the present principles of hospital financing seem frozen in subterfuge, at least on the Eastern seaboard:

1. Overcharge paying patients to pick up county, city, state, and federal responsibility for the indigent sick — money which should come at least partially from a broad tax base;

2. Contain the rising costs of hospital care by giving less money to the hospital, leading to the inevitable downward spiral of financial starvation already the lot of the Boston City Hospital and the JMH.

This story is being told all over this country. Recently a book has been written which concerns itself with the inhumanity of a city hospital long neglected by the politicians *and* the medical profession: the Jefferson Davis in Houston, Texas, a teaching hospital used by Baylor University. [32]

We have been discussing inpatient hospital care. Outpatient services have received even less attention and much less money, and soon urban teaching hospitals are going to have to charge and collect what such service costs. Note what the problem is in Philadelphia, as reported by the *Philadelphia Inquirer:*

A noted Philadelphia surgeon warned City Council on Monday that the city's private hospitals are losing $17 millions a year and unless they get financial relief, including a substantial increase from the city, they may have to close their outpatient clinics.

I. S. Ravdin, executive vice president of medical affairs, University of Pennsylvania, told City Council's Budget Committee that indigent outpatient and emergency care accounted for $7,500,000 of the loss. The city now contributes $1,600,000 a year for this service. [33]

THE COST FOR ONE PATIENT FOR ONE DAY

An analysis of the cost per diem of a patient at the MGH should be rewarding. Perhaps we can then answer two questions: (1) *who* should be paying for certain costs in teaching hospitals, and (2) are *all* the costs justified in teaching hospitals?

The cost per patient per day at the MGH in 1964 was $50 (figure rounded off). A glance at Table V will show "routine" (room and board) costs of $30.99 and ancillary costs of $19.11 per day. Careful examination of the breakdown of these costs should make it clear why the cost is $50 a day in the urban teaching hospital. It has always been a source of concern and frustration to me that almost everyone knows the figure $50 a day, but almost no one knows

123

TABLE V. Massachusetts General Hospital, analysis of inpatient costs per day, fiscal year 1963–64 (total, $50.10).

Room and board (routine costs)

Administration (executive, accounting, purchasing, personnel, admitting, information, telephone, credit, dispatch, employee fringe benefits)	$1.99
Operation of plant (utilities, elevators, parking)	0.56
Plant maintenance (maintenance shops–building repairs)	0.61
Laundry and linen expense	1.61
Building service (housekeeping)	1.03
Food	4.85
Services (chiefs of service and house staff)	2.48
Nursing service	11.10
Nursing education	2.26
Drugs and medication (for which no separate charge to the patient is made)	1.21
Medical and surgical supplies (gauze, dressings, adhesives, thermometers, instruments, enamelware)	1.71
Medical records	0.33
Maintenance of personnel	0.21
Social service	0.59
Depreciation	0.45
Total	$30.99

Ancillary expense

Operating rooms		$ 5.54
Anesthesiology		
Professional salaries	$1.38	
Other costs	1.09	2.47
Radiology		
Professional salaries	1.61	
Other costs	1.29	2.90
Laboratories		5.26
Electrocardiograms		0.31
Physical medicine		0.41
Medical supplies (for which a separate charge to patient is made. This includes I.V. solutions)		1.31
Drugs (for which a separate charge to the patient is made)		0.91
Total		$19.11

a single item of the total expense. Arguments for containing hospital costs usually take place against a background of inadequate information or ignorance. Since 11.6¢ on the dollar of cost represents the hotel function, the MGH hotel cost on this per diem rate is roughly $6.00, a fairly good hotel room rate to say the least!

"Cost" represents the raw or actual cost of taking care of the average patient for one day. Our average *charge* per day is roughly $10 greater because of losses due to free service, public agency (welfare) reimbursement (in 1964 we were allowed a maximum of $40.79 per day for welfare patients, nearly $10 below our costs), Blue Cross contractual losses (comprehensive contract holders pay costs and did not share our net unreimbursed free care), bad debts, and employee allowances, in the proportions shown in the following list.

Losses necessitating charges greater than actual costs

Free service	$ 3.60
Welfare losses	3.20
Blue Cross contractual loss	2.00
Employee allowance and W.C.A.	1.00
Bad debts	0.20
Total	$10.00

The average charge of $60 per day *is* paid by direct paying patients and those covered by Blue Cross co-insurance contracts (on the routine charge but not the contract for ancillary services) and commercial insurance plans. They are assuming the responsibility which has not been borne by existing state and federal welfare programs and which is not shared by Blue Cross comprehensive contract holders and cannot be met by existing endowment income and United Community Services allocation. If our charges were paid equally by all the patients or their third-party representatives, then our charges would be reduced for all and our cost would equal our charges for all involved. One segment of the hospital's population would then be relieved of paying for another segment, an obligation which should be met ultimately by the use of tax dollars. I see no reason why a sick person should be his sick brother's keeper. I might also add that it is our intention to have one set of ancillary charges for all areas of the hospital and to do away with all the social and professional differences among the groups receiving ward, semiprivate, and private care. Our ancillary charges will also be reduced gradually to cost, and any added charge will be confined to the routine side of expense where it can be identified easily and defended.

ELEMENTS OF COST

Turning to Table VI, we see that certain elements of the total cost have been stripped away from the routine and ancillary areas where they reside, to give a new per diem cost of $40.66. These elements have been chosen because they are the most controversial in the minds of public and some segments of the profession alike. Who should, or better, *might* pay these costs?

Nursing School. All would agree that the patient should pay for the service he receives from the student nurse, but not all would agree that he should pay for the time spent in education. The problem may be solved by time, what with the expansion and increasing popularity of collegiate nursing programs and the accelerating decline of the hospital "diploma" schools. Time alone is not the answer, however, for our hospital schools still supply two-thirds of all the nurses in the United States. Many college graduates will become faculty members, visiting nurses, and admin-

TABLE VI. Massachusetts General Hospital, inpatient costs per day with controversial items removed.[a]

Room and Board (fiscal 1963–64 total)	$31.00	
Nursing school	− 2.26	
Residents' maintenance and salaries	2.48	
Depreciation	0.45	
Adjusted total		$25.81
Ancillary (fiscal 1963–64 total)	19.00	
Anesthesiology salaries	− 1.38	
Radiology salaries	1.61	
Pathology salaries	0.36	
Residents in O.R.	0.17	
Other laboratories (M.D. salaries)	0.63	
Adjusted total		14.85
NEW TOTAL PER DAY		$40.66
Analysis of new total		
Nursing service		11.10
Drugs		1.21
Laboratory technicians		4.55
Food		4.85
Operating rooms		5.50
Radiotherapy (other than M.D.s)		1.29
Anesthesia (other than M.D.s)		1.09
Miscellaneous (EKG, physical therapy, social service, medical records, etc.)		5.07
Total (minus hotel cost)		$34.66

Leaving hotel cost approximately $6.00/day

a Professors and chiefs of service salaries included in the routine expense, partly in residents' expense and also in the salaries of anesthesiologists, radiologists, and pathologists. The MGH paid salaries of $1,366,148 and Harvard gave $374,350. In addition, through research grants from all outside sources, the MGH paid $1,877,075 (not a patient expense) and Harvard paid $678,198.

istrators and will not be available for nursing hospitalized patients. Therefore hospital schools must continue. Who will pay for them? The only alternative to support by the hospital's only earning asset — the patient — is state and federal support through departments of education. There are certain objections to this, and I just smile when the state's welfare man says "We shouldn't pay this — why don't you get it from the department of education?" or "You should go to Washington and get the HEW to pay this cost." I am ready, willing, and able to crusade, but the present methods of financing must prevail until a new and better method is ready to function. If both these sources of support should fail, the universities would have to assume the full responsibility. They probably will in time, but by evolution and *not* revolution. It is probable that equitable sharing of the fixed responsibility will develop, as it has between university and teaching hospital in the area of medical students and house officers. The university supports the medical student; and the teaching hospital, the graduate doctor in training. Similar programs will develop as regards nursing students and graduate nurses. The recently enacted federal legislation for nursing schools should help considerably by giving money for construction of new facilities and for scholarships. For the time being, the hospital's patients will continue to pay for the nursing school.

House Staff. The cost of the interns and residents is now allowed as a reimbursable expense by all paying agencies. Paradoxically, the state's Welfare Department has challenged this too, asking why it should pay for doctors in training. Welfare officials argue that the teaching hospital must have welfare patients and that the house staff keep the patients for their own educational needs, citing longer stays and higher utilization of ancillary services such as laboratory tests and radiological procedures. The Commonwealth of Massachusetts, in implementing the Kerr-

Mills Bill, has ruled that no professional fees will be paid to local doctors if the welfare patient lives within fifteen miles of a teaching hospital. Even the Massachusetts Medical Society, in challenging the legality of the fifteen-mile limitation, stated at a Hearing on Welfare Practices in April 1964 that "the patient's stay in the teaching hospital is likely to be more prolonged than in the local hospital." [34]

Such attitudes are particularly annoying. The welfare patients and the medically indigent in general are older and sicker than is our private patient population of active wage earners. The former are frequently referred to us from a local hospital. It is largely aged people who cannot pay their medical bills who occupy our ward beds. They stay longer for both medical and social reasons. Multiple system disease and poor or inadequate after-caring facilities result in higher utilization of ancillary facilities and longer stays, respectively. We have completed a factual study which proves this point. I speak from personal experience as a visiting physician who continues to teach medicine when I say that the house staff makes the error of discharging these patients too soon rather than too late. As soon as the diagnosis is made and management instituted, the young physician-in-training wants another new, *acute* challenge.

Part, but not all, of the higher ancillary utilization can be explained by the patients' age and medical condition. However, unbridled enthusiasm for tests and total belief in medical technology have led us astray and leave us highly vulnerable to the outside paying agents. Medical faculties have not taught by rewarding restraint and thoughtfulness in the use of tests but usually have condemned the house officer when he missed one determination. How often have we, as teachers, been given the

values for BUN, CO_2, Na, Cl and K when a specific gravity
of the urine was not done or was glossed over? Is it not
possible that medicine can be taught by explaining why
certain tests are not needed, rather than by resigning ourselves to a trial-and-error method on the part of the house
staff? In some teaching hospitals today, $80 worth of tests
are done on anyone and everyone with abdominal pain
and vomiting. Responsibility and attention to medical
costs is needed here, and the public has a right to demand it.

Certainly, the cost of the house staff must be borne by the
hospital's patients. Salaries are still far too low for this
group, who could after all be licensed in most states and
charge their own fees. The average cost of $2 over a
twenty-four-hour period (actually $2.48 for inpatients)
provides for the most careful medical examination in the
world today and for continuous care come what may. It
is entirely justified and allows the hospital to give the
highest quality of care obtainable. The AMA agrees with
this, but it and the Blue Shield that it controls do *not* want
to pay for this cost; nor do most of the other third-party
payers! It is a logical and easily defended hospital cost.
It will continue to rise until medical house staff are paid
decent, living wages.

Professors' (Full-Time) Salaries. Here again, and for similar reasons, the cost of the patient care element of our
full-time clinical chiefs can be justified as a hospital expense. The medical school should generally pay that part
of the total salary which relates to the individual's university function of teaching and research. The hospital's part
of the salary is given for the service function of patient care
and the necessary administrative responsibility surrounding it. Obviously there is no formula here, for on a given
day with a given patient the professor may be simultane-

ously carrying out research, teaching, and patient care. Research generally is paid for by research funds, and its financing is kept entirely separate in our budget. During 1964 the MGH paid salaries of $1,366,148,* exclusive of house staff, and the Harvard Medical School paid the same individuals roughly $374,350. I see no reason why the MGH's part shouldn't be paid by the hospital's patients.

Depreciation. Some have argued that the segment of the population unfortunate enough to be sick and hospitalized should not have to pay what in our hospital amounts to over 45¢ a day so that tomorrow's patient can have an adequately maintained plant and facilities. I have heard medical school deans say that the federal government should pay for this; and, happily for many hospitals, the Hill-Burton Act will provide now for the renovation and alteration of urban hospitals. Unfortunately, the cost of depreciation was never included in the charge structure of many hospitals, while others have been unable to earn it, covering their deficits by not spending and diverting the money allocated in the budget for depreciation. More often than not, as we have noted, it has been used to cover unreimbursed free care. There are no successful businesses run this way in this country, and it is incredible that hospital boards of trustees, who are usually successful businessmen, have not championed the cause of earning and spending depreciation in hospitals. Many hospitals, particularly large urban complexes, can survive now *only* if federal money is made available to renovate their plants. Again, however, one could argue that the entire community and not just the hospitalized segment should main-

---

* In addition, the MGH paid M.D. salaries of $1,877,075 and Research Fellows $944,954 through research grants, mainly from the N.I.H. Harvard also paid an additional $678,198 to our doctors through research grants.

tain their hospitals through one of two mechanisms: private philanthropy (which has not been adequate to date) or the tax dollar. For the present, those hospitals which can must continue to include depreciation in their charges; and when the depreciation isn't earned, the money must be made available by fund drives or Hill-Burton allocations and it must be *spent on schedule*. I believe that the patient should pay for depreciation, as he is the main reason that the plant and equipment are depreciating.

Salaries for Anesthetists and Radiologists. Radiologists in particular (and the AMA in general) have been opposed to a salaried arrangement with hospitals. If we were to remove the salaries of radiologists, anesthesiologists, and pathologists, we could reduce our ancillary rate by $4.15, but I believe that these departments are vital services and should be well organized on a basis which is not subject to the ability of the patient to pay.

From the standpoint of the hospital director, the removal of all these controversial elements from the hospital's cost of caring for the sick might make life much easier. Just imagine how much simpler it would be to explain a cost of $40.66 instead of a charge of $60.00. Further, if we removed the cost of nursing service, we could reduce our daily cost to $29.56. As shown in Table VI, we arrive finally at a hotel cost of $6.00 per day. We could then compare this rate to a one-night stay in a hotel. The comparison would be very favorable for hospitals. We would be relieved of rationalizing the cost of and the need for student nurses, house staff, teaching in general, depreciation, radiologists, anesthetists and pathologists and even graduate nurses. We could confine ourselves to the simple task of comparing our cost with that of the local hotel, which people can understand easily, for it is the only comparison they are able to make rationally at the present time. Personally, I am delighted that the public wants to hear and that we are in a position to tell why costs are high and what exactly patients are getting for their money. The gain for medicine and hospitals in an enlightened public is incalculable.

REGIONAL PLANNING

No discussion of social responsibility is complete without a discussion of medical care planning. The past thirty years have seen repeated formal attempts to organize, distribute, and utilize health services rationally, [35] whether it be in the form of the Bingham Associates Fund of New England in 1931, the Hospital Survey and Construction Act of 1946 (the Hill-Burton Act), the development of regional planning councils, or Public Law 89–97 ("Medicare") and the Heart Disease, Cancer and Stroke Law of 1965. Involvement by government in regional planning has increased markedly as private and local initiative has been judged inadequate to the task. State as well as federal involvement is increasing. In New York, legislation was passed in 1964 (the Metcalf-McCloskey Law) which provides for a State Hospital Review and Planning Council which acts as an advisory body to the State Department of Public Health, although final decisions rest with the State Department of Social Welfare. The State Council receives applications from seven regional councils for New York State for approval of such things as reimbursement rates and permission to build new facilities. Recently the Folsom Committee, appointed by Governor Rockefeller to study rising hospital costs, succeeded in effecting certain amendments to the public health and social welfare laws which (1) place all responsibility for new construction and supervision of health facilities under the Commissioner and

Department of Public Health, and (2) add the *equipment* (and equipping) of such facilities to the definition of construction, and therefore subject them to final approval by the state. [36] The legislation introduced as a result of the Folsom Committee recommendations was passed in record time, attesting to the importance that the public and its political representatives place on insuring responsible planning for health facilities.

The expansion of medical knowledge and the rising cost of medical care demand effective regional planning (1) to organize, distribute, and utilize health services rationally for the better care of the sick and injured as well as the prevention of disease, and (2) to contain unnecessary expense by the avoidance of duplication or underutilization of costly machinery and building of unnecessary facilities. We run into difficulty immediately as we argue the virtues and defects of a planned, centrally controlled society versus the spontaneously adjusted, unplanned, "laissez-faire" condition. Rational behavior in the activities of intelligent, mature men occurs when their goals are quantifiable, unambiguous, and internally consistent. The values from which the goals are derived must not be in conflict. The laissez-faire society satisfied these conditions for the ultimate goal of all economic activity, that is, profit. [37] Unfortunately, the ends of medicine are not readily quantified (for example, what do "freedom from *dis-ease*" and "social, psychic and somatic health for all" mean and how can they be evaluated and measured?); contain many ambiguities (such as the special requirements of the doctor-patient relationship, and the allegedly detrimental effect of prepayment and administrative controls designed to facilitate the free access of patients to doctors); and are not always internally consistent (for example, providing high-quality care and better services for *all* the people while simultaneously containing or reducing costs). Furthermore, central planning does not guarantee more rational decisions. We must also accept the uncomfortable fact that what may seem rational planning today can be altered overnight by the inexorable advance of medical science and technology even though social and medical values remain the same.

Recognition of the limitations of central planning does not alter the fact that responsible men should attempt to rationalize their activities. Expanding knowledge, rising expectations, and rising costs demand that medicine provide a more effective social technology. As regards the development of facilities in the community, it is quite clear that there is, *first,* better service to be given and, *second,* less capital and operating expense to be incurred if the beds, operating rooms, and technical facilities are used maximally (which, except for cultural difficulties, might demand a seven-day work week). This statement applies most clearly to obstetrical and pediatric facilities and to those needed for the cobalt bomb, open-heart surgery, and organ transplantation. After that, even the most avid planner recognizes that effective regional planning results in increased capital expenditure to improve existing facilities and build new ones, and furthermore, that there are local community needs and initiatives which central planning cannot understand and may ignore or even stifle. The hazards of "equality," that is, culturally safe mediocrity achieved through weakening the strong in order to improve the weak (which, though unintended, is guaranteed by the "rules and regulations" of central authority), must also be guarded against. Restricted state and federal budgets and inadequate reimbursement formulae for hospital care have contributed to a nation-wide degeneration of plant and facilities — and adequate money in the future for the funding of depreciation may be the single most important aspect of effective regional planning over the long run.

A wide body of useful knowledge now exists about regional planning; [38–40] and some voluntary regional planning councils which include the local financial establishment have operated with marked success. State departments of public health have also planned well for community facilities. Unfortunately, such community service and planning is foreign to most medical schools, their faculties and students; and schools of public health have long since been cut off from the mainstream of medical education. Resistance to regional planning comes not only from religious and trustee groups, but even more important, from the medical profession itself. It is to be hoped that the Heart Disease, Cancer and Stroke Law with its directed assistance will succeed in fostering rational regional planning, where the Hill-Burton program of equality for all has failed at least in part.

The first problem becomes one of selecting a politically viable planning unit. One must be able to encompass the problems of a given region in terms of population, cultural characteristics, and political controls. A strongly motivated lay board of directors, with the active participation of the medical profession and a staff adequate to the task, is absolutely essential. The medical profession does not suffer lay control gladly, but one must remember that the expert sacrifices the wisdom of common sense and the impartiality of nonvested interest to the intensity of his experience. The secretary of defense is not a general of the army for obvious reasons.

One must have clear-cut values and goals for planning in the development of community health facilities, goals and values which can be stated as follows.

SOCIAL RESPONSIBILITY

1. The first principle and the principal goal is to improve service in the care of the sick and the prevention of disease. Any saving of money is a secondary gain, which may not always be achieved as community needs are uncovered which may require more personnel and additional capital expenditures.

2. Local initiative must be encouraged by the active participation and understanding of *all* segments of the community.

3. The irrational as well as the rational needs of patient and physician must be considered by the planning board, for although planning for facilities can be rationalized, the behavior of doctors and patients is not always predictable or rational. The intensely personal nature of their relationship cannot be ignored, nor should it be subjected to the starvation of bureaucratic controls. Detailed knowledge of the sociology of doctors and patients is needed if our facilities are to be used wisely.

4. The university must play a central role in planning. Its rich intellectual resources must be made available to the planning group. Hopefully, the elements of medical care planning will become a part of the medical school curriculum so that the physician can ultimately contribute to change through planning rather than resist it through fear of the unknown. The relevant disciplines centered in schools of public health should be integral parts of the medical school curriculum, and the rationalization of the whole spectrum of health services should be an on-going area of research and teaching within the university.

5. While planning for facilities, the problems of manpower must also be considered. New machinery and new facilities such as hospitals, nursing homes, and public health units are useless and even harmful if technical and professional help is unavailable or inadequately trained.

JOHN H. KNOWLES, M.D.

The provision of a healthy environment for those who care for the sick is important. They should not be depressed by dismal or inefficient surroundings built by poorly trained individuals. The recruitment of such critically needed manpower is the responsibility of all of us and cannot be delegated to a central authority alone. Doctors can learn much and help considerably in influencing a larger number of each new generation to enter the medical world and work effectively once there; administrators and trustees play a crucial role in their management policies in retaining manpower; local and federal political representatives can help through detailed understanding and support of better and more expensive hospital care while encouraging utilization of lower cost, after-caring facilities. The Eighty-Ninth Congress has shown this understanding through the Medicare and Heart Disease Laws.

For the future, technical facilities will become increasingly important in the application of new knowledge in the care of the sick. Historically, plant and facilities have received short shrift at the hands of city, state, and federal authorities, and the subdivision of the tax dollar has always found the hospital at the lowest end of the pole in terms of operating expense and replacement monies. In this regard, one page of history is worth a volume of logic, to paraphrase Louis Brandeis. In the era of expanding scientific and technological advance, the teaching of medicine and service to the community cannot be carried out in inadequate existing facilities, to say nothing of the increasing capital expenditures necessary to establish the new medical technology. The building of facilities per se does not guarantee full utilization of new knowledge if planning is inadequate and manpower is deficient. Trustees, community leaders, medical profession, and medical faculty must be able to plan rationally so that a public *and* private

138

SOCIAL RESPONSIBILITY

system of medical care can combine to advance the frontiers of medicine. If responsible planning on a private, local basis fails, then our political representatives will turn to the more distant and more centralized federal planning — and local initiative and responsibility will wither, to the detriment of our national effort to match need and action to produce a better and healthier society.

CONCLUSION

Our American society has accepted the concepts of social welfare, and although it is still ruggedly individualistic, it looks increasingly to the federal government for help in the solution of the social and economic problems of an increasingly complex and specialized country. As the representatives of the organized consumers of medical care have grown in influence and power — the unions, the Blue Cross and commercial insurance companies, state and federal welfare representatives *and* the politicians — so the organized voices of the medical profession, the AMA and the AAMC, seem to have lost the quality of timely response. Increasing numbers of legislative commissions are inevitable in this era of rapidly rising hospital costs, and organized medicine will be assaulted with paradoxical demands. The unions fight to keep the insurance premiums of their members down while simultaneously demanding unionization of hospital employees to gain better pay. Which way do they want it? Three-fourths of the insurance premium goes into employee salaries. Raise salaries, raise premiums. There is no other way! Welfare departments feed hospitals three-quarters money and one-quarter sawdust while the politicians wait for the hospital scandal because of inadequate money (to maintain adequate standards), for which their predecessors were responsible. The maintenance of rising standards necessitated by increasing medical knowledge demands increasing amounts of money, and it is impossible today to have optimal medical care without adequate funds.

Present and past investigations in Boston and New York have pitted the public and the politicians against the Blue Cross and the hospitals on the basis of rising and "extravagant" costs. In New York City, Ray Trussell, the Commissioner of Hospitals, has investigated the lowering of standards, particularly in the city-owned hospitals, and has been given the necessary authority *and* money to remedy the situation. At the same time, a new study commission has been created to study the meteoric rise in Blue Cross premiums. In Boston, ink was barely dry on the report of one legislative commission when another was created for much the same purpose. From what we have read in the newspapers, Miami has been indulging in the same activities related to the Jackson Memorial Hospital. It will be interesting to see what happens in Houston and Philadelphia.

With the growth of Blue Cross, the hospital has acquired a buffer between it and the public. The political assault starts with the Blue Cross and then stops with the hospital, which thus effectively protects the medical school and its interests and serves as its buffer. Inevitably, medical school deans and university presidents are going to be asked directly to explain their solutions to the problems of rising costs, rising expectations and their fulfillment, and the absolute needs for medical education (including hospital facilities). Interest in teaching and research must be matched by interest in the social service of medicine. Good medical care cannot be demonstrated in inadequate technical facilities and plant, nor can it be distributed effectively by those who ignore the major problems of the community.

Some of those who graze in upland academic pastures

in the foothills of Mount Olympus believe that socialized medicine will solve our financial problems. A glance at some of the results should bring them up short — specifically, what has happened to the Boston City Hospital, the Jackson Memorial Hospital, and Houston's Jefferson Davis, under the heel of politically determined priorities on the tax dollar. If we don't fight now for the money to provide the highest standards and the best facilities, will we be any more effective when the money is being doled out from Washington and local city, county, and state departments? The financing of medical research is one thing, but the sordid history of financing urban hospital facilities is quite another and does not breed optimism. Medical school deans recoil from the realities of money and standards in hospitals by taking refuge in the higher abstractions of educational methodology. Yet they know that patients, money, and standards are needed to teach medical students.

Who *is* protecting the interests of the teaching hospital? Organized consumers are indulging in short-term self-interest, as their main concern seems to be "Keep the premiums down!" They seem to have lost the concept of "It is *our* hospital and as a vital institution in our community we should understand it and help to improve it." Medical staffs still view the hospital as their host and their workshop. They have generally resisted collective action to help reduce hospital costs, such as effective participation in regional planning, closer attention to admitting and discharge policies, and willingness to accommodate themselves to the needs of the institution (for example, operating in the afternoon and on Saturdays, planned vacations to maintain an even census, exerting a staying hand on overzealous house officers busily ordering multiple tests, and so on). Medical school deans and their faculties are preoccupied with a curriculum which has not undergone

JOHN H. KNOWLES, M.D.

significant change since the Flexner Report in 1910 and which leaves the student to his own devices as regards the social "science" of medicine. Hospital directors criticize their staffs for lack of interest in the hospital and its over-all problems, and yet make no efforts to communicate the problems clearly and succinctly to the staff and to enlist their help, based on understanding of the problems. Politicians make hay with the present apathetic confusion and the lack of any clear, persistent voice from the medical profession except "Make no change — the problems will solve themselves!" The voice from the voters is clear, even if unrealistic: "Keep the standards up and the costs down!"

On this battlefield of disarray, every vested interest is fighting, but only a few understand or want to understand the vital interrelationship among all these interests on a long-term basis. The world is full of specialists and cries out for generalists. The summit is crowded with politicians and bereft of statesmen. The orbit of patient, doctor, hospital, medical school, Blue Cross, state and federal welfare department, union leader, "healthy" public and political representative, must be closed and strengthened if the best medical care is to be available to the citizens of this country. Indifference or lack of responsiveness and understanding on the part of any of these vital elements will weaken the whole purpose of medicine and jeopardize the highest attainment of its goals.

The *teaching hospital* must educate its staff to the present socio-economic problems that it faces and enlist its help in solving them. It must develop careful cost accounting and then be able to explain and justify the detailed costs to the staff, the public, and the third-party payers. It must expand its ambulatory clinic facilities and experiment with new functional arrangements for the delivery of medical care and the prepayment for such care. [41] The

Blue Cross and other insurance companies must agree to full payment for ambulatory services. The hospital interest should bring pressure to bear for a change in the medical curriculum so that a more enlightened product can bring about change, using the hospital as a social instrument instead of as a convenient host. The hospital must be willing to assess the quality of its care and to control its proper utilization. It must make constant attempts to contain costs, but much of this work will be done by its enlightened and responsible medical staff. It must involve itself in regional planning on a continuing basis.

The *medical school* must descend from Mount Olympus and come to grips with the social problems of medicine and face the public and its representatives. A good way to start is with a more detailed understanding of medical care financing and the delivery of care as seen from the teaching hospital. The day is fast approaching when inadequate distribution and financing of medical care will adversely affect the quality, the teaching, and the very purpose of medicine. Medicine is firmly established as a biological science but has never achieved its full potential as a social science. This can happen only if the medical curriculum is changed to provide for the continuing influence of sociology, economics, social history, and public health interests through the four years of medical school. Planning for the medical needs of the community must become a university interest. If the university is committed to the teaching hospital as a *social* as well as an educational instrument, it must encourage social research. Medical care research must develop and influence the curriculum.

Our university hospitals plow through these troubled waters with what might be called "la belle indifference," sailing under the flag of biological science. Schools of public health, which do concern themselves with the social, economic, organizational, and distributional problems of medical care, have long since been splintered off from the medical school and the undergraduate medical curriculum, and the intellectual shutters of the medical student have been closed involuntarily to this expanding body of information. Departments of preventive medicine too often confine themselves to the campus and are rarely seen on the firing line of the hospital; they are given only a fleeting moment in the curriculum to cross the arid desert of epidemiology and biostatistics.

The university hospital continues to see what is interesting while leaving what is difficult to the community — its other hospitals, struggling physicians, political representatives, *and* voters. The outside expert — the politician, the social historian, the economist, the social psychologist — has today a clearer view of the problems of medical care than the experts of the inner sanctum — the medical faculty and its products: the practicing physicians and medical faculty of tomorrow. The practicing physician, isolated from the major socio-economic problems of scientific medicine in medical school and the university hospital and generally confined to biological science for his intellectual development, has also not realized the major aim of education: to be, as Lionel Trilling said, "at home in and in control of the modern world." [42] If, as John Dewey said, education is the fundamental method of social progress and reform, how much social progress and reform has been brought about by the medical profession and the present medical curriculum?

I am firmly convinced that the last half of this century will be notable for its attention to the social problems of medicine and that triumphant solutions will equal biologic discoveries in excitement and importance. The timely response of hospitals, the AMA, the AAMC, and most important, the universities, is long overdue, and silence will *not* be golden on these issues. Teaching costs must be defended, hospital facilities must be maintained; and, with the force of an enlightened public, the increasingly powerful arbiter of social progress — the politician — will understand and make long-term decisions designed to encourage and protect the two most important institutions in medical care today — the hospital and the medical school.

This is medicine's clarion call. The public craves balanced information in depth from the medical establishment, which it is not receiving. The balance of power is tipped to an unenlightened public, and our political representatives are making their decisions on this basis. Medicine must help to shape its own destiny. The option will be removed if it ignores its social responsibility. A sound relationship based on mutual understanding between teaching hospital and medical school can only serve to strengthen the work of both. The sinews of such a relationship are the proper identification of their respective functions and their common goals and the appropriate administrative framework within which to achieve these goals.

NOTES

KNOWLES: INTRODUCTION

1. Bertrand Russell, *Has Man a Future?* (Simon and Schuster, 1962), p. 126.
2. J. S. Bruner, *On Knowing: Essays for the Left Hand* (Cambridge: Harvard University Press, 1962), p. 160.
3. W. H. Stewart, "Education for the Health Professions," address delivered at the White House Conference on Health, November 3, 1965, General Session. By permission of the author.

GLASER: THE TEACHING HOSPITAL AND THE
MEDICAL SCHOOL

1. W. B. Wood, Jr., *From Miasmas to Molecules* (New York: Columbia University Press, 1961), p. 1.
2. Abraham Flexner, *Daniel Coit Gilman: Creator of the American Type of University* (New York: Harcourt, 1946).
3. G. P. Berry in *Report of the First Institute of Clinical Teaching*, edited by H. H. Gee and J. B. Richmond (Evanston: Association of American Medical Colleges, 1959), p. xxiii. Reprinted with permission of Association of American Medical Colleges.
4. Abraham Flexner, *Medical Education in the United States and Canada*, A Report to the Carnegie Foundation for the Advancement of Teaching (New York: Carnegie Foundation, 1910; reprinted in 1960).
5. *Ibid.*, p. 240.
6. J. E. Garland, *Every Man Our Neighbor* (Boston: Little, Brown & Co., 1961), p. 5.
7. *Ibid.*, p. 6.
8. W. F. Norwood, "Medical Education and the Rise of Hospitals. II. Nineteenth Century," *J.A.M.A.*, vol. 186 (1963), p. 1008.
9. S. Flexner and J. T. Flexner, *William Henry Welch and the Heroic Age of American Medicine* (New York: Viking Press, 1941), p. 136.

10. H. H. Merritt, "Medical Care, Education and Research. Present Day Medical Education and the Medical Center Concept," *N.E.J.Med.*, vol. 271 (1964), p. 1194.

11. J. H. Knowles, "The Social Conscience and the Primary Function of the Hospital Viewed in Historical Perspective," *Pharos*, vol. 26 (1963), p. 67.

12. J. E. Dietrick and R. C. Berson, *Medical Schools in the United States at Mid-Century* (New York: McGraw-Hill Book Co., Inc., 1953), p. 140.

13. John Steinbeck, *Travels with Charley* (Bantam Books, Inc., 1963), p. 107.

14. Niccolo Machiavelli, *The Prince* (translated by L. Ricci, revised by E. R. P. Vincent; New York: The New American Library of World Literature, 1952), p. 49.

RUSSELL: SURGERY IN A TIME OF CHANGE

1. Wilfred Trotter, "Commemoration of Great Men," *British Medical Journal*, vol. 1 (1932), p. 317.

2. Celsus, *De Medicina* (with an English translation by W. G. Spencer; Loeb Classical Library, Harvard University Press, 1938), vol. I, Book VII, p. 1.

3. V. F. Blehl, ed., *The Essential Newman* (Mentor-Omega, The New York American Library, 1963), p. 173.

4. W. H. Ogilvie, *Surgery Orthodox and Heterodox* (Springfield, Ill.: Charles C Thomas, 1948), p. 36.

5. E. D. Churchill, "The Surgeon and the University," address delivered October 15, 1954, at the Centennial of Queen's University, Kingston, Ontario.

6. John Davy, "Choosing Your Career at 14," *Observer* (London), December 13, 1964.

7. W. C. Rappleye, "Emerging Patterns of American Medicine," Alpha Omega Alpha Lecture, Columbia University College of Physicians and Surgeons, New York, May 13, 1964.

8. G. K. Dunlop and J. G. Freymann, "Utilization of Private Patients in Surgical Education," *J.A.M.A.*, vol. 184 (1963), p. 930.

9. R. V. Lee, "Preparation of Practitioners of the Future," *J. Med. Education*, vol. 40 (1965), p. 70.

EBERT: THE DILEMMA OF MEDICAL TEACHING IN AN AFFLUENT SOCIETY

1. J. K. Galbraith, *The Affluent Society* (Boston: Houghton-Mifflin, 1958), pp. 1–2.

NOTES: EBERT

2. N. I. Bowditch, *History of the Massachusetts General Hospital* (Cambridge, 1872), p. 3.
3. *Ibid.*, p. 4.
4. *Ibid.*, p. 8.
5. *Ibid.*, p. 9.
6. *Annual Report of the Trustees of the Massachusetts General Hospital*, 1873, p. 37.

KNOWLES: MEDICAL SCHOOL, TEACHING HOSPITAL, AND SOCIAL RESPONSIBILITY

1. Alexis de Tocqueville, *Democracy in America*, Knopf ed., vol. II, p. 128.
Parts of this paper were delivered at the Second Institute on Medical Center Problems of the Association of American Medical Colleges in Miami, Florida on December 9, 1964 and at a Panel Meeting of the Task Force on Economic Growth and Opportunity of the U. S. Chamber of Commerce in Washington, D. C. on December 10, 1964; and have been published in *J. Med. Ed.*, vol. 40, part 2 (November 1965), p. 167 and the *Harvard Medical Alumni Bulletin*, vol. 40 (Christmas, 1965), p. 2.
2. R. M. Titmuss, *Essays on the Welfare State* (New Haven: Yale University Press, 1959), pp. 133, 134.
3. "Medical Care in the United States," U.S. Dept. of Health, Education and Welfare, Public Health Service, March 1961.
4. *New York Times*, Sunday, October 4, 1964, p. 50.
5. W. M. Dixon, *The Human Situation* (London: Edward Arnold, Ltd., 1957), p. 173.
6. E. C. Hughes, "Professions," *Daedalus*, vol. 92 (1964), p. 655.
7. H. L. Smith in E. H. Jaco, *Patients, Physicians and Illness* (Glencoe, Ill.: The Free Press, 1958), pp. 469–470.
8. Editorial, "Challenge to Responsibility," *J.A.M.A.*, vol. 190 (1964), p. 60.
9. *New York Times*, Sunday, February 16, 1964, p. 2.
10. "Report of the President," John and Mary R. Markle Foundation, 1962–63, pp. 10–11.
11. J. H. Knowles, "Freedom Versus Responsibility" (editorial), *The Pharos of A.O.A.*, vol. 27 (1964), p. 54.
12. David Riesman, *Abundance for What?* (Garden City: Doubleday, 1964), p. 303.
13. *Ibid.*, p. 306.
14. *Ibid.*, p. 308.

15. D. A. Clark and C. G. Sheps, *et al.*, "Study of Affiliations Between Medical Schools and Teaching Hospitals. A Preliminary Report," Evanston, Ill., A.A.M.C., 1962.

16. D. A. Clark and C. G. Sheps, "On the Administration of University Teaching Hospitals," *J. Med. Ed.*, vol. 39 (1964), pp. 527–530.

17. *Ibid.*, p. 530.

18. Letter to the Editor from Dr. Robert Williams, *N. Eng. J. Med.*, vol. 271 (1964), p. 1121.

19. J. H. Knowles, "The Balanced Biology of the Teaching Hospital," *N. Eng. J. Med.*, vol. 269 (1963), pp. 401–406, 450–455.

20. "The New Power of the Financial Executives," *Fortune*, vol. 65 (January 1962), p. 81.

21. *Ibid.*, p. 85.

22. C. I. Schottland, *The Social Security Program in the United States* (New York: Appleton-Century Crofts, 1963), chap. 4.

23. L. Engel, "The Ills of 'Maintown Hospital,'" *New York Times Magazine*, Sunday, November 26, 1961, pp. 98, 100.

24. *Ibid.*, p. 43.

25. Boston Redevelopment Authority Report, "Reviewing Boston's Municipal Facilities," 1963.

26. L. S. Reed and D. P. Rice, "National Health Expenditures: Object of Expenditures and Source of Funds, 1962," *Soc. Sec. Bull.*, August 1964, pp. 11–21.

27. *New York Times*, Saturday, October 24, 1964, p. 19.

28. "Source Book of Health Insurance Data 1963," Health Insurance Institute, N. Y.

29. H. M. and A. R. Somers, *Doctors, Patients and Health Insurance* (Washington: The Brookings Institution, 1961), p. 295.

30. "Blue Cross Blues," *Wall Street Journal*, June 5, 1964, p. 1.

31. J. H. Knowles, "Report of the General Director," *One hundred and fiftieth Annual Report of the Trustees of the Massachusetts General Hospital for the Year 1963*, pp. 50–53.

32. J. deHartog, *The Hospital* (New York: Athaneum, 1964), p. 337.

33. *The Philadelphia Inquirer*, Tuesday morning, November 17, 1964, p. 29.

34. Memorandum from Massachusetts Medical Society presented April 11, 1964, p. 4.

35. John H. Knowles, ed., *Hospitals, Doctors and the Public Interest* (Cambridge: Harvard University Press, 1965), p. 317.

36. Marion B. Folsom, personal communication, June 1965. See also State of New York, Governor's Committee on Hospital Costs,

"Summary of Findings and Recommendations," April 9, 1965, Marion B. Folsom, Chairman.

37. Harry Eckstein, *The English Health Service* (Cambridge: Harvard University Press, 1958), p. 266.

38. "Profiles in Planning: A.M.A. Directory of Health Facility Planning Agencies" (Chicago, 1965).

39. "Areawide Planning: Report of the First National Conference on Areawide Health Facilities Planning, American Medical Association" (Chicago, 1965).

40. "Areawide Planning for Hospitals and Related Health Facilities," U.S.P.H.S. Publication No. 855, July 1961; and Publication No. 930-B-3, September 1963.

41. J. H. Knowles, "The Medical Center and the Community Health Center," *Bull. N. Y. Acad. Med.*, vol. 40 (1964), pp. 713–742.

42. Lionel Trilling, "Commitment to the Modern," *Harvard Alumni Bulletin*, vol. 64 (July 1962), p. 739.

INDEX

151

MEDICAL LIBRARY
NORTH MEMORIAL HEALTH CARE
3300 OAKDALE AVENUE NORTH
ROBBINSDALE, MN 55422

Knowles, John H.   WZ80
The teaching hospital   K73t

16422

MEDICAL LIBRARY
NORTH MEMORIAL HEALTH CARE
3300 OAKDALE AVE. NORTH
ROBBINSDALE, MINNESOTA 55422